Dear L

Enjoy my

Book!

Marlin.

Ultimate PULMONARY WELLNESS

A New Book by

Dr. Noah Greenspan

DPT, CCS, EMT-B

Doctor of Physical Therapy
Cardiovascular and Pulmonary Clinical Specialist
NYS Emergency Medical Technician-Basic

Edited by Mark W. Mangus, Sr.

BSRC, RRT, RPFT, FAARC

Foreword by Norma MT Braun, MD

Pulmonary Wellness & Rehabilitation Center
10 East 38th Street, New York, NY 10016
212.921.0214
www.PulmonaryWellness.com
noah@pulmonarywellness.com

ISBN: 978-1-54390-843-5 (print)
ISBN: 978-1-54390-844-2 (ebook)

This publication was made possible by the Nora and Roger Gimbel Family Fund.

If you would like to support the Pulmonary Wellness Society in their mission to provide free educational opportunities for those living with pulmonary disease, you can make a tax-deductible donation at www.PulmonaryWellness.com/Society.

For My Grandma Peppie,
the kindest, most generous person I have ever known.

For My Brother, David, who understood instinctively that
there will never be a shortage of people in the world
that need our help.

It is not the critic who counts, not the man who points out how the strong man stumbles, or where the doer of deeds could have done them better. The credit belongs to the man who is actually in the arena, whose face is marred by dust and sweat and blood; who strives valiantly; who errs, who comes short again and again, because there is no effort without error and shortcoming; but who does actually strive to do the deeds; who knows great enthusiasms, the great devotions; who spends himself in a worthy cause; who at the best knows in the end the triumph of high achievement, and who at the worst, if he fails, at least fails while daring greatly, so that his place shall never be with those cold and timid souls who neither know victory nor defeat.

– Theodore Roosevelt

TABLE OF CONTENTS

FOREWORD BY NORMA MT BRAUN, MD

Dr. Noah Greenspan has dedicated his life, his energy, and his creativity to helping people with various cardiopulmonary disorders lead more symptom-controlled and enjoyable lives. I have personally known Noah for more than 15 years and he is truly a unique healthcare advocate and wellness innovator. In *Ultimate Pulmonary Wellness*, he has written a self-help treatise for patients to better understand the origins of their breathing limitations and to learn how to perform better in all spheres of life.

Noah has written each chapter as a stand-alone entity so the reader can choose what they read and when, refer back to it as many times as they desire and continue to come away with a better understanding of his or her individual issues as they relate to shortness of breath or *dyspnea*. He writes in a style that is easy to read and understand, describing the origins of cardiorespiratory symptoms, their associated manifestations; and practical methodologies to address them, along with compassion and humor.

From anatomy and physiology to symptom genesis and pathophysiology; how to ask your physician for specific information; the ins and outs of breathing and respiratory disease, exercise, how to nourish the only body you have and a precise medication usage guide to optimally enhance your lung function, Noah makes it clear that *you* are his focus, with individualizing each strategy to *your* specific needs being central to the program.

This comprehensive treatise is a very valuable and handy field guide for anyone who wants to live a happier, more productive, and symptom-free life with respiratory disease.

Yours truly,

Norma MT Braun, MD

Clinical Professor of Medicine
Icahn School of Medicine, Mt. Sinai Health Systems
Mt. Sinai St. Luke's – Mt. Sinai West
Department of Medicine
Pulmonary/Critical Care/Sleep Division

EDITOR'S NOTE BY RESPIRATORY THERAPIST LAUREATE, MARK MANGUS

There are a number of books available focused on providing information, education and assistance for those who endure the difficulties of living with a chronic lung disease. As is evident in other efforts in this realm, success in writing in a manner that is both easily understood; and also captures succinctness and accuracy in content treads a fine and sometimes treacherous line. Many falter, either mischaracterizing facts, misstating them, or otherwise failing to accomplish that goal. Noah has managed to succeed where many have faltered, presenting much information while also keeping his writing style light, extremely readable and fun. One will find themselves chuckling, perhaps without warning or expectation, as they traverse the pages of ***Ultimate Pulmonary Wellness***.

As one with many years' experience writing on both a professional, technical level and translating the technical to understandable patient language, I know firsthand how difficult is the task to tread that line of which I speak. In the process of editing this book, and in composing my contribution to its text, I have learned much from Noah in the art of presenting that information in both an easy reading form and a more fun and light-hearted style, much appreciated by readers—some of whom have been so kind to provide to us their honest and unpretentious feedback along the way.

On a personal note, I want to say that I am honored and proud to have had the good fortune to be a part of the genesis of this book, which Noah and I are confident will be a great source of hope and help for those who read it. Other than perhaps those who have worked by Noah's side for these many years of contemplation, consternation, and crafting of this book, I am among those few who truly understand the labor of love and commitment this work represents. Noah, I am grateful to know you, to experience your infectious spirit, collegial counsel, friendship and your genuine compassionate concern for those we serve, along with greater humanity.

Sincerely,

Mark Mangus, Sr., BSRC, RRT, RPFT, FAARC
Chronic Lung Disease Management Specialist

INTRODUCTION

"The best time to plant a tree is twenty years ago. The second best time is now." **– Chinese Proverb**

If you are reading this book, it is more than likely that you or someone you know have at one time or another, experienced the sensation of being short of breath due to respiratory disease, cardiovascular disease or both. Shortness of breath (SOB), also known as *dyspnea* (pronounced disp-nee-uh) or *air hunger* (pronounced air hun-ger), can be all encompassing and has the potential to undermine every aspect of your life, from the magnificent to the mundane.

There are few sensations in life that are as absolutely terrifying as not being able to catch your breath. In fact, most of us will do absolutely everything in our power to avoid that sensation at all costs, even at the expense of things we love, such as going to the theater, visiting with friends and family; even everyday activities such as taking a shower or grocery shopping; even having sex. Shortness of breath can deliver a tremendous blow to our self-esteem as well as our overall quality of life, but I don't have to tell you these things. You already know them because you or someone you know has experienced them firsthand, and there are few greater teachers in life than firsthand experience.

My mission in writing this book is to teach you that for the overwhelming majority of people, being diagnosed with a respiratory disease is *not* a death sentence and your situation does *not* have to be hopeless, nor should it be. In fact, there are *many* things you can do to *minimize* your shortness of breath as well as to *maximize* your overall health and quality of life.

My mission in writing this book is *not* to sell you a bill of goods promising a quick fix or cure for your disease or an overnight solution to your shortness of breath. You didn't get here overnight. You're not getting out overnight either. I'm also *not* suggesting that managing your disease will be easy. It will not. I repeat. Managing your pulmonary disease will *not* be easy. *But*...if you follow the suggestions in this book, even some of the suggestions, some of the time, I promise you that you will begin to experience small (and in many cases, not so small) but noticeable improvements in your daily life, whether it be less shortness of breath, the ability to do more of the things you love, increased energy levels, or an improvement in your overall sense of well-being.

This is not something I *think*. This is something I *know* from firsthand experience because I have seen it work time and time again over the course of my 25-year career as a cardiopulmonary physical therapist, taking care of patients just like you or someone you love.

Many of the suggestions in this book will work for *many*, if not *most* people reading it. However, it is important to understand that when it comes to patient care and people in general, all of us are different and therefore, need to be treated as individuals. As such, there will always be exceptions to the rule that will require some adjustments or "tinkering" with the methodology.

SOB or *dyspnea on exertion* (DOE) is by far, the single most common presenting symptom of respiratory disease and almost always the symptom that causes people to seek medical attention *and my assistance*. However, it is extremely important to note that shortness of breath can also be the consequence of many conditions besides respiratory disease; ranging in severity from the very serious, like cardiovascular disease, anemia, or renal disease; to the more benign, but still important-to-address conditions like gastro-esophageal reflux disease (GERD) or deconditioning due to inactivity (i.e. being out of shape); or it could be related to something else entirely.

My point in telling you this is that I don't want you to make any assumptions or self-diagnoses as to the cause of your shortness of breath, without being sure that there aren't other contributing factors that can potentially be harmful to you if left untreated. With that in mind, it is absolutely essential that your physician perform a comprehensive workup of your symptoms before beginning any meaningful course of treatment or undertaking any significant lifestyle change *such as cardiopulmonary physical therapy or pulmonary rehabilitation.*

SOB can range in severity from barely noticeable to all encompassing. At times, you may not even be aware of your symptoms while at others, they may stop you dead (or at least, completely breathless) in your tracks. Depending upon where you are, what you happen to be doing, even who you happen to be with at the time, you may attempt to minimize or make light of your symptoms. You may even tell yourself (and others) little white lies such as: "I'm getting old" or "I'm out of shape" or "it's not a big deal." But, you know darn well it is. When I hear people use phrases like "it's not a big deal," I am reminded of that famous river in northeast Africa called: "the Nile." Denial, get it?

Typically, most people first begin to experience shortness of breath at high levels of exertion, during activities such as stair climbing or walking uphill. In New York City, the three things patients complain about most are climbing subway stairs, walking up the city's many hills and inclines and running *or walking quickly* for the bus; or what we not-so-affectionately like to call "the NYC Pulmonary Triathlon."

Human nature dictates that when we start to experience a certain symptom; any symptom, whether it be shortness of breath, chest pain, back, hip or knee pain; or any other physical (or emotional) distress, we will typically find ways to alleviate or minimize our discomfort; either by modifying the activity that causes us to be symptomatic (e.g. walking more slowly or taking more frequent rest breaks), or by avoiding the activity altogether (e.g. taking a different route or driving, instead of walking uphill or climbing the stairs).

Therein lies *at least part* of the problem. The fact is, once you start to avoid the activities that cause you discomfort (whether they be stair climbing, walking uphill or running for the bus), all of the muscles that you use to perform these activities (including, most importantly, the heart; as well as the respiratory and skeletal muscles), become weaker and more deconditioned. And when muscles become deconditioned, they don't perform as well or use oxygen as efficiently. As a result, you begin to experience shortness of breath at lower levels of activity, and eventually, start to avoid those lower level activities as well and so on and so on. This is what is known as the "*Dyspnea Cycle.*"

In addition to the muscles themselves, all of the body systems that are involved in performing these activities also become less efficient and when these systems don't operate as well, guess what. You become *even shorter* of breath at *even lower* levels of activity and in turn, start to avoid *those* activities as well, beginning the cycle all over again. *Sound familiar?*

At the Pulmonary Wellness & Rehabilitation Center (whether in person or via the Ultimate Pulmonary Wellness Webinar Series, Ultimate Pulmonary Wellness Facebook Group, or this book), our goal is to help you break this cycle in three ways. First, we teach you more effective breathing techniques designed to increase your awareness of and give you greater control over your shortness of breath. Second, we will teach you how to exercise, both aerobically (e.g. treadmill, exercise bike, upper body ergometer) and anaerobically (e.g. strength training), so that your body becomes stronger and more efficient at using oxygen and you become less short of breath.

Last, but definitely not least, we will educate you about the various lifestyle factors that play a role in how well or how poorly you breathe, so that you can begin to *reverse* your shortness of breath as well as any other limitations or modifications you've had to make and that have wreaked so much havoc in your life.

With this principle in mind, my purpose in writing this book is *not* to give you a complex list of instructions or fancy protocols that are difficult to understand and virtually impossible to follow. Instead, my goal is to present you with a wealth of information that my patients and I have found to be both successful and practical over the past 25 years.

Again, each person is different and every situation is unique. Therefore, not all things will work for all people. However, my hope is that this information will help guide you and your healthcare team in determining which tools and techniques will work best *for you* and which ones won't be as helpful, or not helpful at all.

As I mentioned earlier, there are few greater teachers than firsthand experience. I am proud to say that the overwhelming majority of what I have learned about pulmonary disease (and its most effective management) has come from my patients. I have been extremely fortunate to be exposed to great instructors and brilliant mentors throughout both my formal education and my professional career but by far, it has been my patients that have been my most instrumental teachers.

I earned my Bachelor of Science in physical therapy in 1992 from the *State University of New York Upstate Medical University* in Syracuse, New York, with the help of professors like Susan Miller and program director, Chuck Meacci, who truly *forced* me to reach my full potential; pushing me way past my own limits, albeit, in an extremely compassionate and nurturing way, mind you; much like what we do with our patients. In fact, I am positive there were many times that *they* believed in me more than I believed in myself, also much like with our patients.

I earned my Doctor of Physical Therapy in 2006 from Dominican College in Blauvelt, NY. I am also board-certified by the American Board of Physical Therapy Specialties in Cardiovascular and Pulmonary Physical Therapy as well as a New York State Emergency Medical Technician (EMT-B).

I was fortunate to have "grown up" professionally at the New York University (now Langone) Medical Center's Rusk Institute of Rehabilitation Medicine in New York City. I put the words "grown up" in quotes because there are many that might argue the validity of that statement. *Anyhoo*, my experience at NYU allowed me to develop my clinical skills and figure out not only what I wanted to be doing with myself, but also what I didn't want to do. I had incredible mentors including doctors, Horacio Pineda, MD, a beloved physiatrist and pioneer of Rusk's cardiopulmonary rehabilitation program and Mariano

Rey, MD, who was not only a brilliant cardiologist but also a mad tactical visionary, always seeing the big picture quickly and knowing how to get things done within a complex medical and political environment.

In 1995, when I was still only 24 years old, these two giants of medicine took a chance by giving me the opportunity to become the chief physical therapist of the Center's cardiac and pulmonary rehabilitation programs; changing my life forever; despite the fact that the rest of the medical center let out a collective gasp of "Noah?" That was long before texting but if it weren't, I am sure there would have been a flurry of 3-letter responses like OMG, SMH, WTF...you get the idea but it was Drs. Pineda and Rey who gave me my shot and for that, I will *always* be grateful.

I've also had the great fortune to be surrounded by amazing colleagues whom I both respect and trust implicitly. Marion Mackles is without question one of the greatest cardiopulmonary and chest physical therapists, a*nd friends* that I have ever known. Marion and I met in 1994 and have been working together for more than two decades.

In 1998, she was just crazy enough to join me in opening the Pulmonary Wellness & Rehabilitation Center. At that time, we spent a lot of nervous hours staring at the walls as we waited for our first patients. Most people predicted we'd remain in business for about 3-6 months but I'm proud to say that we're still going strong nearly 20 years later.

I was also incredibly blessed to have met one of the greatest personal influences of my life, Lawrence Joseph Virgilio, in 1994. Larry and I crossed paths while we were moonlighting on the weekends at Beth Israel Medical Center in NYC. A short time later, he signed on as the weekend physical therapist at NYU's cardiac rehabilitation program.

Larry was a Fireman with Manhattan's elite Rescue Squad 18 in the West Village and also a Senior Physical Therapist at the Pulmonary Wellness & Rehabilitation Center. To this day, I have never encountered someone who routinely developed as natural a rapport with patients, and people, in general, as Larry. I mean, this guy would meet a patient once and for weeks after (months, even), that patient would still be asking how he was doing or to send him their regards. After Marion and I left NYU to open the Pulmonary Wellness Center, I was both thrilled and honored to hear Larry's voice on the phone asking if he could join us.

The kind of things I learned from Larry cannot be taught in books; things like how to stay (or at least appear) calm in an emergency, how to reassure patients even in the most serious circumstances and also, the importance of not getting caught up in the small stuff that life can throw at you. Larry was a true gentleman and a gentle man but believe me. He could also be as tough as nails when he needed to be.

I still have a newspaper clipping in my desk with a picture of Larry leaning over the side of a building hanging on to a construction worker with one arm after the guy's scaffold collapsed. Larry worked at the Pulmonary Wellness & Rehabilitation Center until September 11, 2001 at 10:28 AM, when he died in the North Tower of the World Trade Center during the single greatest rescue effort in the history of the FDNY.

Another person I am thankful to have worked with is one of my former students, Greg Sweeney, also an outstanding cardiopulmonary physical therapist, who at the time of this writing is the program manager of NYU's cardiac and pulmonary rehabilitation program. Over the years, I have watched Greg grow into one of the finest cardiopulmonary therapists and educators in the field. In 2013, Greg and I developed and co-taught a Continuing Medical Education (CME) course called

"Cardiovascular of the Rehabilitation Patient," a primer on the implications of cardiovascular system and heart disease on rehabilitation.

Of course, I also have to credit my parents, Sherry and Mel Greenspan, and my sisters, Erika and Farrah, who have always supported me in whatever endeavor I chose to undertake, as well as my brother David, who understood instinctively that there will never be a shortage of people in the world that need our help.

I also have to pay the greatest homage to my Grandma Peppie, who was by far, the kindest; most generous and most supportive person I have known…ever. I can honestly say that without her, I wouldn't be the person I am today. In her eyes, I could do no wrong. If someone asked her who did something, she would be like: "I don't know who did it but I know who didn't do it, *my Noah*."

Since opening the Pulmonary Wellness & Rehabilitation Center in 1998, we have conducted over 85,000 exercise sessions and at this point, I can confidently say that we pretty much have it down to a science. For that, I am grateful for the loyalty and dedication of my team including Marion, Akua Adu-Labi, Aastha Joshi, Wai Chin, Patricia Rocco, Melina Francis, and Caroline Kelley, as well as many others that have spent some time with us over the years; as well as the many physicians, who have honored us with the privilege of caring for their patients.

One such physician is Dr. Norma Braun, MD, who has honored me with her foreword to this book. I have been hearing legendary tales of Dr. Braun's unconventional methods for decades; including her spending hours on end sitting by her patients' bedside while they are weaned from a ventilator or going back to their birth in reviewing their medical histories. When I say unconventional, I mean this with the highest possible respect and admiration although it doesn't really do justice to this medical giant whose compassionate patient care is equally matched by her tenacity in getting to the bottom of each patient's problem; and then stopping at nothing to address each problem one by one. Gregory House, MD has nothing on Dr. Braun.

I want to thank Mark Mangus, Sr., BSRC, RRT, RPFT, FAARC, who I refer to as the respiratory *therapist laureate*. Few clinicians have the absolute wealth of knowledge and experience that Mark does. In addition to spending time with us at the Center, Mark has been an invaluable contributor to this book and co-author of the chapter on medications.

I also want to thank Nicole Speletic, Ph.D., a gifted writer and deep thinker, who added a great deal of texture to the fabric of this book, Rena Miller, my Co-Admin of the Ultimate Pulmonary Wellness Facebook Group, who is great at helping to "keep the main thing the main thing," and Sylvia Johnson, who was a late-game editing *blessing*.

Finally, last but never, ever least, I must once again acknowledge my many patients, who are by far the driving force behind who I am as a clinician and who I strive to be as a human being. It is through these symbiotic relationships, with the very people who come to me for help; allowing me to participate in their lives and getting to know them through their disease; that I am constantly learning about myself and continuing to grow, both professionally and personally.

In sharing our collective experience with you, I hope to give you a direct link to the greatest source of information about your disease, in an effort to help you avoid some of the same pitfalls that others before you have had to deal with. One thing that I can tell you for certain is that even more gratifying than trial and error; is trial and success, especially when it comes to my patients.

The good news is that the overwhelming majority of the information being passed on to you has come directly from the source: *other patients*. They are the true *experts* in the field, who have experienced many of the same struggles as you *and* found ways to overcome them, even when it seemed like all odds were against them and *you can too*. It is my hope that by putting our collective knowledge and experience together in one comprehensive, yet easy to understand "bible" for pulmonary patients, you will have at your disposal, a wealth of options to choose from, and that you too, will be able to experience your own little slice of "Ultimate Pulmonary Wellness."

Nothing in the world gives me greater satisfaction than helping people breathe better, to feel well instead of sick, and to truly live their lives instead of watching it pass them by from the sidelines. A big part of that involves clearing up confusion about their disease and dispelling myths and misinformation (of which, there is a lot), an unfortunate but not uncommon byproduct of today's fast-paced healthcare environment.

In some ways, the Internet can be one of the best sources of medical information, but in others, it can also be one of the most detrimental, not to mention, terrifying. For one thing, information on the Internet is not always completely accurate or current. Often, it's not even remotely accurate, and sometimes, people discover far more than they ever wanted to know, often completely out of context and without a proper filter or guide to help them separate fact from fiction.

That's what I'm here for. I wrote this book to help remedy that precise situation and to help clear up any confusion you may have regarding your disease (or at least point you in the right direction). *Ultimate Pulmonary Wellness* is meant to be an infinitely and intimately useful guidebook covering the medical, behavioral, and lifestyle issues of not just living; but *living well* and *thriving*, despite your pulmonary condition.

On this journey, I will cover some of the basics, taking you on a quick tour of the *functional* anatomy and physiology of the respiratory system as well as some key components of the cardiovascular system. I will also guide you through the diagnostic process, explaining some of the many tests and procedures you may undergo, as well as some of the more commonly used medical practices and interventions.

We will also go through what I believe are the five key components of Ultimate Pulmonary Wellness: Medical, including finding the right doctor, taking the right medications, and *taking them properly*; Exercise, Nutrition, Stress and Anxiety Management/Meditation; and Prevention of Infection.

As for smoking, you *know* what you have to do. As Nike says, "*Just Do It*" (or in the case of smoking, just *don't* do it). That includes cigars, pipes, hookah, and "e-cigarettes."

In this book, you will find useful, proven tips, as well as images, charts and worksheets that you can use to record notes and track your progress. I've also included a glossary of key terms because there's nothing more frustrating than when medical professionals use fancy jargon or complicated medical terms without a corresponding "Gibberish to English" dictionary.

I'm so thankful that you have decided to read this book and to take the first steps in making your life better. This means more than simply not being short of breath, or learning how to live with your disease and its associated symptoms. Instead, it means setting out on a path to truly becoming your best self and to achieving your own state of *Ultimate Pulmonary Wellness.*

I wish you all the best in life and hope that if you're in New York City, you'll stop by the Center. We play great music, sing karaoke, and have amazing art on the walls. We have beautiful fish and the greatest dog named *Monkey*. We have *a lot* of laughs and do everything we can to spoil our patients rotten. We also happen to get great results!

CHAPTER 1

SHORTNESS OF BREATH

"If you can't breathe, nothing else matters."
– American Lung Association

As I mentioned in the introduction, when people begin to experience shortness of breath or dyspnea on exertion (DOE), they either find ways to modify the activities that cause them discomfort or they simply avoid them altogether. While this may seem like the safest and most reasonable course of action, decreasing your activity will actually worsen the situation, causing you to become weaker and weaker over time, until even life's simplest tasks, like showering or getting dressed, can become difficult thanks to *that miserable SOB (shortness of breath).*

Let's use stair climbing as an example. In New York City, subway steps are definitely *not* built for comfort. Rather, they are designed for efficiency, which in New York City means "space-saving." As a result, they are usually longer, higher, and steeper than the stairs in most people's homes or even those you might encounter in a restaurant or movie theater. Add to this scenario, a mob of type-A New Yorkers during rush hour, and the situation more closely resembles the running of the bulls than a daily commute. Patients frequently tell me that they don't take the subway any more because they can no longer climb the stairs. Instead, they take the bus or taxi, or Access-A-Ride, (but that's a whole 'nother story, altogether).

Again, using our stair-climbing example, think about how much less activity a person will get if they switch from taking the subway to taking the bus. Let's say they usually commute to work five days per week and have two flights of stairs going to work and two flights coming back home. That's 20 flights of stairs per week—80 flights per month—and nearly 1000 flights per year.

It isn't hard to imagine that if you climb 1000 fewer flights of stairs this year than you did last year, your body will naturally (or more accurately, *unnaturally*), become less conditioned, and you will likely experience an increase in your shortness of breath. Incidentally, these negative adaptations to inactivity can happen even if you don't have a pulmonary disease.

Now, here is a concept that is very important to understand. The inability to climb stairs can be affected by many factors including shortness of breath, cardiovascular disease, muscle weakness or fatigue. It can even be caused by anxiety, which, incidentally, is both increased by shortness of breath and increases shortness of breath (*another vicious cycle we want to break).*

As you become more deconditioned, your body does not use oxygen as efficiently. As a result, you then start to feel short of breath at lower levels of activity. Then, you start to avoid *those* (even lower-level) activities, and so on and so forth. Again, this is called *the dyspnea cycle* or *dyspnea spiral* and as I mentioned earlier, our goal is to help you break that cycle by teaching you more effective breathing techniques—and teaching you how to exercise *most* effectively every time, so that your body becomes more efficient at using oxygen and you, less short of breath.

For many people, their symptoms can get so bad that the activity doesn't seem possible or worth the effort any more. Depending upon where you live and the resources available to you, this scenario can drastically limit the things you can do, the places you can go, and the people you can see.

Some of my patients are able to map out the city by where there are steep (or in some cases, not so steep) inclines or hills. Others can map out the city based on where there are places to sit down and rest, and still others, by the availability of public restrooms. They take the easier routes whenever possible and avoid hills like the plague. But as you might have guessed, all of the muscles that they use to walk uphill become deconditioned, and they now start to feel short of breath at even lower levels of activity (e.g. walking on flat surfaces). *Sound familiar?*

There is also another important possibility that you (and your doctor) should consider. Believe it or not, it is completely possible that your shortness of breath could be the result of something else altogether. Patients come to me all the time that can't understand why they're more short of breath. "Nothing has changed," they protest. That's when I start my interrogation. I inquire knowingly as to whether there have been any changes in their medications, exercise regimen, weight, and etcetera, etcetera.

"Oh, yeah. I have gained a little weight," they say. To which I say: "How much? "About 25 pounds," they say (or 30, or 40, or more). To which I say: "So, you've gained 25 pounds and think nothing's changed?"

Let me put this in perspective for you: 25 pounds is the equivalent of two bowling balls. Try carrying two bowling balls around with you all day, every day, for a while. I am pretty sure that you will get tired more easily, have more difficulty climbing stairs, and yes; feel more short of breath.

We'll discuss the subject of weight in greater detail in the nutrition chapter, but my point in introducing it now, is to illustrate that there are many factors besides the lungs and the respiratory system that contribute to breathing and consequently, SOB

Patients often report feeling more short of breath, despite no significant worsening of their lung function on Pulmonary Function Test (PFT). Conversely, patients may report an improvement in their symptoms, without a corresponding improvement in their PFT. What this tells us is that there absolutely, positively have to be other factors besides pulmonary function that affect how well or how poorly we breathe.

At the Pulmonary Wellness & Rehabilitation Center, our goal is to help patients break this "dyspnea cycle" by teaching them more effective breathing techniques and by exercising them most effectively (*i.e. vigorously*), so that their bodies get better at using oxygen. We also *educate* our patients about their disease, medications, the benefits of exercise and eating healthy, managing stress and anxiety, and the pitfalls of cigarette smoking and inactivity. I truly believe that in the overwhelming majority of cases, an educated patient will be a healthier (and happier) patient.

A common principle in medical ethics is "*Primum Non Nocere.*" This phrase comes from the Latin, meaning, "*First, do no harm.*" At our Center, patient safety is our first, second, and third priority. We believe in a "no-setback" approach to cardiopulmonary physical therapy and rehabilitation and when it comes to patient care, I don't like surprises. That's why everything we do at the Center is done under fully monitored conditions.

As our patients exercise, they are "telemetrically monitored", which is a fancy way of saying that they wear an electrocardiogram (ECG), so that we can continuously monitor their heart rate and rhythm during exercise. Their blood pressure and oxygen saturation are each measured in

5-minute increments. Again, our patients' safety is our first, second, and third priority.

The beauty of this type of monitoring system is that we can be confident in making adjustments to our patients' programs—not just on a daily basis, but even within each individual workout, allowing us to ensure not only their safety, but also that they are receiving the maximum benefit from each and every session. This methodology is the real secret to our success—*and of course, the karaoke.*

Please feel free to share this information with your healthcare team and please be sure to get your doctor's go-ahead before beginning *any* exercise program or implementing *any* lifestyle change. And who knows? He or she may even learn a thing or two that can help their other patients.

Finally, your attitude is essential. I understand that when you feel sick, it can be difficult to focus on being shiny, happy and positive. However, constantly focusing on your illness or all the things you *can't do* can have a profoundly negative impact on your health and wellbeing. Throughout this book, I will be guiding you and sharing methods that will help you work your way back to wellness, so that your actions and thoughts can begin to have a profoundly *positive* impact on your health and wellbeing—in other words, your life. Don't worry about the starting line. For now, think of yourself as the healthiest you can be *today*...and then get ready to become even healthier.

CHAPTER 2
THE RESPIRATORY SYSTEM

"Breathe! You are alive."
– Thich Nhat Hanh, Zen Buddhist Monk

KNOW THYSELF!

It never ceases to amaze me how many people I meet, who are living with a chronic illness, often for years, who have little or no knowledge about the biological system involved, let alone the disease itself and its impact on their bodies and their lives. Please understand that it is *not* my intention to present you with a doctoral-level dissertation on the respiratory system (and I'm pretty sure you don't want one).

However, when it comes to dealing with a chronic illness, a *basic* understanding of the anatomy (structure), physiology (function) and pathophysiology (disease) will go a long way. My hope is that this information will help you better understand your condition, as well as provide you with the necessary vocabulary and context for more meaningful communication with your doctor and other health care professionals. Throughout this book, I will explain how various factors affect your breathing and what you can do to improve not just your breathing, but also your life.

Breathing is "Multi-Factorial"

I tell people over and over again: "*breathing is a multi-factorial process*." What I mean by that is that on any given day, there are a whole host of factors, both internal and external to our bodies that can affect how well (or how poorly) we breathe. Besides just our lungs and the respiratory system, these can include things like proper medication use, activity versus inactivity, the foods we eat (or don't eat), maintaining a healthy weight as compared to being overweight or underweight and managing stress and anxiety effectively; not to mention the possible effects of weather; and other environmental factors that can have either a positive or negative impact on our breathing.

As an example, think about how your body reacts when you step outside on a cold winter day as opposed to when it's hot and humid; or how you feel after indulging in a big meal or having a few too many cocktails. Using temperature as an example, we know that our body functions best at a temperature of 98.6 degrees Fahrenheit. This is why we sweat in the summer and shiver in the winter as our body attempts to cool and warm itself, respectively.

Breathing is Multi-Systemic

Breathing is also *multi-systemic*. Contrary to what many people believe, breathing is not just a function of the lungs and the respiratory system alone. In fact, multiple systems contribute to the act of breathing including the following:

- Neurologic system (brain, spinal cord, and nerves)
- Cardiovascular system (heart and circulation)
- Musculoskeletal system (muscles, bones, joints)

- Endocrine system (glands and hormones)
- Gastrointestinal system (digestion and the digestive tract)

While each system is specialized to perform a different function or set of functions, they are also interconnected, working together; constantly monitoring and adapting to changes in the internal and external environment in an effort to establish a physiologic state of balance known as *equilibrium*.

The net impact of each system will vary depending on the individual and their particular conditions and *co-morbidities*; i.e. other medical issues. Other systems can and will be involved on an individual, case-by-case basis. Therefore, it is essential that you, along with your doctor, investigate and explore all of the factors that *could* potentially be contributing to your shortness of breath.

The Respiratory System

The primary functions of the *respiratory system* are to deliver oxygen (O_2) to the body and remove carbon dioxide (CO_2) and other waste products of metabolism. At the most basic level, when you take a breath, O_2 molecules enter the lungs and cross into the bloodstream. This "*oxygenated*" blood is then transported to the heart, where it is pumped to every cell and organ of the body for use as fuel during metabolism.

CO_2 and other metabolic waste products cross from the cells and organs of the body into the bloodstream. This "*deoxygenated*" blood is then transported back to the heart, where it is pumped to the lungs and expelled during exhalation.

Pulmonary Anatomy and Physiology

Air can enter the body through either the nose or the mouth. When you breathe in through your nose, three important functions are performed. First, the air is *filtered* by tiny hair-like structures; called *cilia*, trapping particles of dust and debris in the mucus membranes. Second and third, the air is also *warmed* and *humidified* by tiny blood vessels called *capillaries*.

From the nose, air continues into the *nasopharynx*, the uppermost part of the throat. When you breathe in through your mouth, air passes through the *oropharynx*, the middle part of the throat. The nasopharynx and oropharynx meet in the back of the throat, or *pharynx*, and continue down through the *laryngopharynx*, the lowest part of your throat and the *larynx* (also known as the voice box).

From the larynx, air enters the *trachea*, or *windpipe*, through the *epiglottis*, a cartilaginous flap that opens during breathing and closes during swallowing to prevent solids and liquids from entering the trachea, airways and lungs.

The *trachea* splits into the right and left mainstem *bronchi*, going to the right and left lung, respectively. The bronchi then continue to divide, getting smaller and smaller, branching into secondary and tertiary bronchi and even smaller *bronchioles*. After approximately 20 to 23 divisions, the air finally reaches the *alveoli*, the tiny air sacs in the lungs where *gas exchange* occurs.

Inhalation

Inhalation is an *active* process, meaning that it requires the active muscular contraction of the *diaphragm*, the *primary muscle of inspiration* (and the *intercostal* muscles) for it to occur. In order for us to take a breath, the brain sends a signal down the spinal cord to the phrenic nerve. When the *phrenic nerve* innervates (i.e. sends an impulse to) the diaphragm, it contracts downward, creating a *negative pressure* in the *thoracic cavity*. It is this negative pressure that causes the lungs to inflate, filling up with air.

When breathing demands increase—as in the case of physical activity or exertion, or in the context of respiratory disease, your body can call on the *accessory muscles*, which include the muscles of the neck, back, and chest, among others, to assist with ventilation.

People with *restrictive lung diseases*, such as *Pulmonary Fibrosis* or *Scleroderma*, have a difficult time with the *inhalation* phase of breathing due to increased stiffness of the lungs. As a result, they have to generate significantly greater force in the respiratory muscles in order to overcome the increased lung resistance.

People with restrictive lung disease often take shallow breaths with less air in each inhalation. As a result, they are forced to breathe more rapidly in order to keep up with the body's ventilation and respiration demands. This is in contrast to people who have *obstructive lung diseases,* who have difficulty in expelling air *out* of the lungs, which I will discuss next.

Exhalation

During quiet breathing, exhalation is a mostly passive process, relying on relaxation of the respiratory muscles, and the natural elastic recoil of the lungs, which causes them to deflate and expel air. Exhalation can also become an active process when the expiratory muscles, particularly the abdominals, contract to actively force air out of the lungs. This *forced exhalation* can be done voluntarily or involuntarily and can occur during strenuous (or not so strenuous) activity, particularly in cases of impaired lung function.

People with obstructive lung diseases, such as COPD do not have difficulty getting air *into* the lungs. Instead, they have a difficult time getting air *out* of the lungs during exhalation. This can be caused by several factors including airway inflammation, mucus or spasm in the airways, a decrease in the natural recoil in the lungs or the destruction of the small airways and alveoli.

Air trapping can also lead to larger (*hyperinflated*) lungs. The more air that is left in the lungs, the less efficient each breath will be in diluting the stale air and sufficiently reducing CO_2. Over time, this can potentially lead to *CO_2-retention* as COPD worsens. This is in contrast to people with restrictive disease, which can lead to smaller (*hypoinflated*) lungs.

In some cases, people can have a combination of both restrictive and obstructive disease, meaning that they have difficulty with both inhalation and exhalation.

Efficiency, Effectiveness and Miles Per Gallon

If you think of your body like an automobile, the efficiency with which your body utilizes oxygen is similar to how many miles you get per gallon of gas (mpg). If your engine is run-down or your oil badly needs changing or your tires don't have the proper amount of air in them, your car will be less efficient and get fewer miles per gallon. The same is true when it comes to your body.

Ventilation and Respiration

The mechanical act of moving air in and out of the lungs; i.e. inhalation and exhalation is called *ventilation.* Ventilation is an *active* process, meaning that it requires the contraction and relaxation of the respiratory muscles, for it to occur.

The chemical exchange of oxygen (O_2) and carbon dioxide (CO_2) between the external environment and the cells of the body is called *respiration* or *gas exchange*. Respiration is a passive process and occurs constantly, regardless of muscle activity or phase of ventilation. In other words, it occurs at the cellular level, during both inhalation and exhalation, as well as during any pauses in between.

While there are many factors involved in how well your body uses oxygen, its overall efficiency is based upon three main factors:

1. How effectively your lungs move air in and out?
2. How effectively your heart pumps blood?
3. How efficiently your muscles utilize oxygen?

If there is a problem in any one of these areas, your body will not be as efficient at using oxygen and you will be more short of breath. For example, if you have a chronic respiratory disease, your lungs will not move air in and out as effectively. If you've had a *myocardial infarction* (heart attack), your heart will not pump blood as effectively. If you lead a sedentary lifestyle, then your muscles will not utilize oxygen as effectively.

If you have problems in more than one area (which is not uncommon), your breathing (and other issues) can multiply. As an example, if you have both heart and lung disease, you will likely have significantly more difficulty than if you had either one alone.

Here is the good news, though, and again, I am completely biased. *But*...in our experience, we have found that the *right* combination and type of exercise and breathing techniques can *significantly* improve the effectiveness of the respiratory, cardiovascular and muscular systems, thereby improving your body's overall efficiency at using oxygen.

In addition, despite a large body of scientific literature stating the opposite, we firmly believe that *under the right conditions*, your pulmonary function can also improve. In the chapter on exercise, I will explain what makes our training methods so different, so effective and what we believe is the key to improving pulmonary function. This will hopefully allow you, the patient, as well as other rehabilitation professionals and programs to benefit from what we at PWRC *know* to be true.

CHAPTER 3

BETTER BREATHING TECHNIQUES

"Give a man a fish, and you feed him for a day; teach him how to fish, and you feed him for a lifetime."
- Chinese Proverb

This saying pretty much sums up my motivation in writing this book as well as my everyday approach to patient care. In fact, every aspect of our program at the Pulmonary Wellness & Rehabilitation Center and the *Ultimate Pulmonary Wellness Webinar Series* is designed to help patients regain control of their breathing and "ultimately," their lives.

By a landslide, the chief complaint that I hear most often is shortness of breath. For that reason, I have decided to place this chapter early in the book because I truly believe that these breathing techniques can have a *major* impact on your life in a relatively short amount of time, giving you greater control over your breathing, reducing your anxiety and allowing you to participate in more of the activities that you want to—in other words, living your life.

As I've already mentioned, for most people, shortness of breath usually begins at high levels of activity such as stair-climbing or walking uphill. To make matters worse, human nature is such that we find every reason under the sun to avoid the activity or activities that cause us shortness of breath. It's like the old joke where a patient says: "Doc, it hurts when I do this," and the doctor replies: "well, don't do that." Similarly, if you get short of breath when you "do that," odds are you aren't going to "do that" very often.

The problem is that once you start eliminating those higher-level activities, all of the muscles you use to climb stairs, walk uphill or run for a bus become deconditioned and when muscles becomes deconditioned, they become less efficient at utilizing oxygen and you then become more short of breath at lower levels of activity. When it comes to SOB, deconditioning is the number one enemy and our number one goal is to help you break this *dyspnea cycle.*

It can be very easy to get caught in the dyspnea cycle of shortness of breath and inactivity, and very difficult to get out. Too often, people avoid the activities that cause them shortness of breath, and for good reason. They're terrified! However, in many cases, this inactivity can actually become more debilitating than their original respiratory impairment. For example, someone stops taking the subway because climbing subway stairs makes them short of breath. Then, they find ways to avoid the blocks with inclines, and before they know it, even walking on flat surfaces causes them to gasp for air.

As another example, many people find showering to be one of the more difficult activities of daily living. *Part* of the reason for this is the increased work of breathing created by upper body exertion. As a result people either shower less frequently, or find alternative methods of bathing. By decreasing the frequency that you shower, the upper body and your respiratory muscles become more deconditioned and consequently, more fatigued at even lower levels of activity.

People find all kinds of reasons to stop doing the things that cause them discomfort. For many people, the biggest one is fear. For others, it's their doctor or other health care professionals telling them to "take it easy." Still, others are waiting until they feel better before resuming their normal activities or beginning a new program. However, without some form of action or intervention, that day may never come. In fact, the longer you do nothing, the more difficult it will be, the longer it will take and the less likely it will be that you actually get moving again.

Keep in mind that increased shortness of breath does not necessarily indicate that your lung function has gotten worse. It is completely possible that your breathing difficulty has gotten worse solely due to inactivity or any one of a thousand other explanations other than a decline in pulmonary function. So, don't throw in the towel just yet.

The good news is that by gaining greater control of your breathing—first, when you are at rest, then during activity, and finally, when you are in distress—your breathing can actually improve and so can your life.

Here is some more good news. In the same way that your condition can spiral downwards under the *wrong* conditions, it can also spiral upwards under the *right* conditions, by implementing positive lifestyle changes. I actually prefer to use the term "life changes," because the term "lifestyle changes" sounds like we'll no longer be "wintering in Miami" or "summering in the Hamptons." And as I've said many times before: "if you want to change your life, you have to change your life."

In the same way that you have gradually eliminated activities that have become difficult for you, you can gradually begin to build those activities back into your daily routine. Again, I'm not saying it will be easy. *Again*, it won't. However, you're definitely worth the effort of trying, and there are definitely strategies and techniques that can help you get moving again. These include things like taking your medications properly, learning more effective breathing techniques, exercising, eating better, learning how to manage your stress and anxiety, and taking steps to *prevent* infection.

Before we go any further, let me be clear about one thing. I am not in any way trying to minimize or downplay the role of the respiratory system in shortness of breath. After all, the cardiopulmonary system is my favorite biological system for a reason. I am also not suggesting that by incorporating these breathing techniques, or by switching from white bread to wheat that all of your breathing problems will go away overnight. They won't. What I *am* saying is that with a little bit of knowledge and effort, you *can* generate positive changes in your body and your life.

This chapter provides you with practical information and simple instructions on how you can regain control of your breathing. My mentor, Dr. Pineda used to say: "Some people wait for things to happen. Some people make things happen and some people say 'what happened'?" Well, get ready, my friends, because we are about to make things happen.

Now, take a deep breath and let's begin.

The Breathing Techniques: Breaking the Cycle

People ask me almost on a daily basis: "what is the best method of breathing?" The truth is that there is not, nor will there ever be, one single breathing technique that works best for all people in all circumstances. Every technique that I teach you will require some personal trial and error and fine-tuning in order to figure out which ones will be most effective *for you* in various situations (as well as which ones may not help you at all).

The first step in breaking the dyspnea cycle is to learn the *controlled breathing techniques (CBT)* that will help you better manage your SOB, or ideally, prevent it in the first place. These include: *Pursed Lip Breathing (PLB)*, *Diaphragmatic Breathing* (*aka abdominal or belly breathing*) and *Paced Breathing*. Although initially, these techniques need to be practiced as separate entities, when I mention controlled breathing techniques or simply, "the breathing", I am referring to using a combination of all three techniques together.

I will also teach you what we commonly refer to as *Recovery from Shortness of Breath*. Based upon my experience, the question that patients want answered first and foremost, is what to do when you simply cannot catch your breath. By far, this is the scenario that people fear most and what I believe prevents many people from being able to break the dyspnea cycle. After all, few things in life are scarier than not being able to breathe or as the American Lung Association says: "if you can't breathe, nothing else matters."

Again, please remember that no single breathing technique will work best for every person in all situations. Also, don't expect *anything* to work immediately or even very quickly. It will definitely take a little time for you to start seeing progress, as well as some personal trial and error. After all, you didn't get into this hole overnight. You aren't getting out overnight either. If pressed for an answer, I would estimate that most people start to feel at least *slightly* better after approximately 3-4 weeks.

Don't let that discourage you. In fact, I think it should be encouraging. My recommendation would be to try out the techniques—all of them—and practice them. And by practice them, I don't mean try them once or twice and pray for a miracle. Try each of them under different circumstances and conditions. Give each technique several chances to work so you really have an opportunity to evaluate what works for you and what doesn't. Trust me. This will be a worthwhile investment of your time and effort. So, please be patient with the techniques and yourself.

Controlled Breathing Techniques

If you have seen any of the UPW webinars or previously participated in a pulmonary rehabilitation program, you may be familiar with some or even all of "the breathing" techniques. Again, please understand that while I will describe each technique separately and you will practice each of them individually, you will actually use all three in concert during exercise and activity. So, when I say, do "the breathing", I am actually referring to all three of these techniques used together for maximum effectiveness.

In addition to teaching you the breathing techniques, I will also show you various ways in which they can be used or modified to suit your own particular needs and abilities. Again, no technique will work for everyone. Just keep in mind that we always have options.

Before we begin, take a moment to observe your "normal" breathing pattern. Are your respirations rapid and shallow or slow and deep? Do you breathe using your abdomen or are you relying on the *accessory muscles* of your upper chest, shoulders, back and neck? By first observing your current breathing pattern, you will start to become more conscious of which muscles and which breathing techniques are working effectively and where you might need to make some changes.

OK. Here it is. The moment you've all been waiting for—time to discuss the actual techniques that will help you break this vicious cycle of SOB and inactivity.

Pursed-Lip Breathing (Pursed-Lip Exhalation)

Pursed-lip breathing (PLB) can help you prolong exhalation, slow down your breathing, and help keep your airways open—all good things. PLB can be used in any position and regardless of whether you breathe in through your nose or mouth. In fact, as an exercise, I would suggest that you practice performing pursed-lip exhalations, breathing in through both your nose AND your mouth (at different times, of course). For the purposes of this exercise, don't worry so much about the timing (yet). Instead, just take note of what it feels like to exhale through pursed lips.

As you breathe in, imagine "smelling the flowers" and as you breathe out through pursed lips, imagine "cooling the soup on a spoon." And please don't blow your soup clear across the room. Just try to cool it off a little. People often use the suggestion, "blow out the candles." However, this is actually the opposite of what we want since the goal of all of the controlled breathing techniques will almost always be relaxed, easy breathing.

As you breathe in, you should feel your abdomen rise. As you breathe out, you should feel your abdomen fall, all the while, keeping your upper chest, shoulders, back and neck muscles as quiet (still) as possible. Try a few cycles and observe the changes in your body. Is your breathing becoming slower and deeper? Are you becoming more relaxed? *If yes, you are doing it right.*

To practice pursed-lip exhalations while breathing *in through the nose*:

1. Sit or recline comfortably in a chair.
2. Relax your upper chest, shoulders, back and neck muscles.
3. Inhale slowly through your nose.

4. Exhale slowly through pursed lips.
5. Repeat

When breathing in through your mouth, imagine sipping slowly through a straw as you breathe in and cooling your soup as you breathe out. Again, as you breathe in, you should feel your abdomen rise. As you breathe out, you should feel your abdomen fall, all the while, keeping your upper chest, shoulders, back and neck muscles as quiet as possible.

To practice pursed-lip exhalations while breathing *in through the mouth*:

1. Sit or recline comfortably in a chair.
2. Relax your upper chest, shoulders, back and neck muscles.
3. Inhale slowly through your mouth.
4. Exhale slowly through pursed lips.
5. Repeat

Diaphragmatic, Abdominal or Belly, Breathing

As I mentioned before, the diaphragm is the primary muscle of *inspiration*. If you've ever watched a baby breathe, you may have noticed that their bellies move in and out with every breath. In other words, they are breathing diaphragmatically. The *diaphragm* is a big, strong muscle, making *diaphragmatic breathing* the most efficient and effective way of moving air in and out of the lungs. In fact, we should all breathe diaphragmatically, whether we have a respiratory illness or not.

This allows the diaphragm to function most effectively, giving it the greatest mechanical advantage while trying to quiet the accessory or secondary muscles of ventilation: those of the upper chest, shoulders, back, and neck. To be clear, it is impossible for us to take a breath without contraction of the diaphragm. However, since most of us have become *most* familiar with the use of "diaphragmatic breathing," I will use this term for consistency. As they say, you can't fight City Hall. Just keep in mind that when we use the term "diaphragmatic breathing," we are really referring to abdominal or belly breathing.

As we get older, factors such as illness, injury, emotional and even social factors can impact our breathing, causing us to become "diaphragmatically incorrect". That was a political joke. As an example, stress and anxiety can cause us to breathe less effectively, taking rapid, shallow breaths and using our upper chest muscles, as opposed to using the diaphragm most effectively. Other factors like respiratory disease, obesity and deconditioning can also impair our breathing, making us work harder with each breath. As a result, many of us have developed some very poor breathing habits. If this sounds like you, it will take a little time and effort to unlearn these habits, but it can be done.

To practice diaphragmatic breathing:

1. Sit or recline comfortably in a chair.
2. Relax your upper chest, shoulders, back and neck muscles.
3. Inhale slowly through your nose. As you inhale, your abdomen should rise as your lungs fill up with air, while keeping your upper chest as still as possible.
4. Exhale slowly through pursed lips (PLB). As you do this, your abdomen should fall.
5. Repeat

Paced Breathing

At this time, we will address the issue of supply and demand by combining the two previously mentioned techniques, *pursed-lip breathing* and *diaphragmatic breathing,* in a coordinated effort, called *Paced Breathing.*

As you increase your activity level, your body requires a greater supply of *oxygen* (air) in order to meet the greater demand of the activity. Therefore, it will be to your advantage to incorporate breathing techniques that allow for the greatest amount of flow, while at the same time, minimizing airway obstruction and air trapping. Again, I would recommend trying them all to figure out which ones will become your "go to" techniques.

The most commonly used pacing pattern is to exhale for twice as long as you inhale. For example, try breathing in through your nose for a count of two and exhaling through pursed lips for a count of four (or 3:6, or 4:8). Breathing in for a count of one and out for two is usually too short and not often effective for most people although sometimes there's no alternative.

To practice paced breathing:

1. Sit comfortably on a chair.
2. Relax your upper chest, shoulders, back and neck muscles.
3. Inhale slowly through your nose for a count of 2.
4. Exhale slowly through pursed lips for a count of 4.
5. Repeat

As you become more comfortable with these techniques, start to utilize paced breathing during your everyday activities, while trying to keep your focus on both pursed-lip and diaphragmatic breathing. Don't worry if you don't get it at first. Learning these strategies is a process and will take some time. To be clear, for most people, this is not a natural breathing pattern so don't expect it to become automatic. It probably won't.

If you have an *obstructive* disease, I would suggest starting by breathing in for two out for four. Then try breathing in for 3 and out for 6, or in for 4 out for 8. If that doesn't work, I would suggest experimenting with lengthening the exhalation, so try in for 2 out for 5, or in for 3, out for 7 or 8.

If you have a *restrictive* disease, I would still suggest starting with in for 2 and out for 4 (or in for 3 and out for 6 or in for 4 and out for 8). If those don't work, I would suggest trying to shorten the exhalation so I would try in for 2 out for 3, or in for 3 and out for 5.

When you use all three techniques together – *diaphragmatic, pursed–lip,* and *paced breathing,* you are doing "*the breathing,*" which I will discuss further in the chapter on activities of daily living (ADL).

Recovery from Shortness of Breath

Finally, last but *definitely* not least, let's discuss a topic called *Recovery From Shortness of Breath*. Now, *please...do not* wait until you are in what I refer to as a "*Code Red*" *situation* before trying to remember these techniques. In fact, the time to begin this training and practice these techniques is when you are comfortable and relaxed (i.e. *now*).

Most of you know this feeling all too well. You can't breathe. Your chest feels tight, and you are suddenly aware of every heartbeat. And as if that's not enough, panic sets in! I can assure you that panic will not help *any* situation. In fact, panic will cause you to breathe even faster and shallower, making the situation worse. Sound familiar? This "*fight or flight*" response can trigger a whole cascade of physiologic responses, few of which will actually be helpful to you.

Let's use stair climbing as an example. Sometimes, just the thought of walking up stairs is enough to increase your anxiety and shortness of breath. As you start to climb, you can feel your breathing becoming more labored and it feels as though your heart is beating out of your chest. You wonder if you might pass out or have a heart attack. Some of you may even think you're going to die.

By this point, you don't know who or what is in control. Is it the shortness of breath? Is it the chest tightness? Maybe it's the anxiety. The only thing you know for sure is that it's definitely *not* you. This is it! ***CODE RED!*** Is it any wonder that people choose to avoid activities that cause *this*? So, what can you do about it?

There are specific actions you can take that will help you to prevent, relieve and recover from shortness of breath. The first (and most important) one is to stop whatever you're doing; second, talk to yourself; third, get into the right position; fourth, start the breathing and fifth, re-assess your situation.

Now, ideally, you would have begun your controlled breathing techniques long before you ever got to this point, but now is not the time for "I told you so."

To practice recovery from shortness of breath:

1. Stop!

First and foremost, stop whatever you're doing that got you in trouble. If it is walking, stop walking. If it is stair climbing, stop climbing. It is highly unlikely that you will be able to regain control of your breathing while continuing the activity that made you short of breath in the first place. Your immediate goal is to put out the fire and at this moment, your supply of air is not meeting the demand of the activity. Therefore, you need to decrease or eliminate the demand by immediately stopping whatever it is you're doing at the time.

2. Talk to yourself.

I'm not talking about some crazy "One Flew Over The Cuckoo's Nest" type of conversation or that long string of expletives that might run through your mind at a time like this. Instead, now is the time to remind yourself that you do know what to do and that you actually have some tools in your arsenal that will help you get out of this jam.

My suggestion of what you might say to remind yourself that you know what to do, would be something original, like "*I know what to do.*" You can also use "*relax,*" "*I am OK,*" "*calm down,*" or whatever phrase or mantra you find most helpful. *And*...the good news is that once you finish this chapter, you actually *will* know what to do. Then it's a matter of practicing the techniques and getting better at them so that you can start to nip that snowball effect in the bud or ideally, avoid it altogether.

Don't get me wrong. Self-talk is not a magic trick that instantly reverses your shortness of breath. Instead, it's a personal call to action, reminding you that you *can* help yourself as opposed to being a passive recipient of all the wonderful gifts that living with a pulmonary disease keeps on giving (sarcasm intended). Given the choice, I will always choose to take action rather than to wait and see what happens.

This is the mindset that you need to adopt when you start to feel short of breath. Remind yourself that you know what to do. Be present. Be in the moment. Be confident. If not, fake it 'til you make it. And if that doesn't work, you might benefit from enrolling in a formal pulmonary rehabilitation program where qualified medical professionals will monitor you and you can develop the skills and confidence you need.

Another thing to be aware of is that people often have a false sense that their heart rate or blood pressure is much higher than it actually is; or that their oxygen saturation is much lower than it actually is. Don't believe everything you think. Finding out that you are OK, even when you may not *feel* OK can be an eye-opening and empowering experience, allowing you to return to activity and get back to living your life again. Confidence can sometimes be the difference between regaining control of your breathing versus a trip to the emergency room.

3. Assume the Position!

Body position can play a tremendous role in how well or how poorly you breathe. There are certain positions that will give you the greatest chance of catching your breath by allowing your diaphragm and your lungs to work more effectively, while others will make breathing more difficult or impossible, like bending over to tie your shoes. By knowing these positions and how to utilize them to your advantage, you will have a much greater chance of minimizing your shortness of breath.

The first part of the position is to bend over. The second part is to fix your upper extremities. In other words, lean forward on your arms.

If you are standing, there are a couple of different ways you can do this. One is by leaning your back against a wall or other stable surface, bending forward at the waist, and placing your hands on your thighs or knees, putting the weight through your arms.

Another option is to lean forward against a wall, table, or other stable surface, bending forward at the waist, and placing your hands or elbows and forearms on the wall or table, again, putting the weight through your arms.

If you are sitting, spread your legs wide apart; bend forward at the waist, and place your elbows and forearms on your thighs or knees, again, putting the weight through your arms.

These positions are effective because they allow the abdominal contents to drop forward, clearing the way for the diaphragm to contract downward more easily. In doing so, the diaphragm, lungs and entire body have the greatest mechanical advantage for breathing, allowing you to move air in and out most freely and effectively.

Open Chain vs. Closed Chain Activity

This is *partially* based on a principle called "*open chain* vs. *closed chain activity*". Using the arms or upper extremities as an example, open chain activities include activities in which the arms are free to move around in space. When the arms are free, the chain is open. When the chain is open, the muscles of the chest, back, and shoulders work to do things like raising and lowering your arms, moving them in and out, or side to side. Raising your arms above your head to get something down from a shelf is an example of an open chain activity.

When we fix the upper extremities (i.e. leaning forward on our elbows or hands) we "close the chain." Closing the chain causes those same muscles of the chest, back, and shoulders to work in their *reverse* action. This helps elevate the ribcage and thorax, improving respiratory mechanics, allowing you to take a deeper breath. This is the reason why many patients with pulmonary disease naturally gravitate toward these positions without ever being taught. When in doubt, assume the position!

4. Begin the Controlled Breathing Techniques.

By this point in your "Code Red" situation (after a brief conversation with yourself), you should already have stopped what you were doing and assumed one of the recovery positions. Now, begin the controlled breathing techniques. Breathe in through your nose and out through pursed lips, breathing in for a count of 2 and out for a count of 4 (or whichever count works best for you), until you fully regain control of your breathing.

5. Reassess and Adapt.

After you have calmed down and regained control of your breathing, re-assess the situation and if necessary, modify the activity that caused your shortness of breath in the first place. Sometimes this can be as simple as walking more slowly or starting the breathing techniques *before* you're in trouble.

To practice recovery from SOB:

1. Stop what you are doing.
2. Talk to yourself, reminding yourself that you know what to do.
3. Assume the position.
4. Begin the controlled breathing techniques.
5. Reassess and adapt.

And there you have it. That's "the breathing." Remember that no single breathing technique will work best for everyone. Therefore, every technique will require some trial and error in order to figure out which ones are most effective *for you*. Breathe easy, my friends!

CHAPTER 4

ACTIVITIES OF DAILY LIVING

"Do what you can, with what you have, where you are."
– Theodore Roosevelt

Supply and Demand

Over the course of any given day, some activities will naturally be more demanding than others. As an example, stair climbing is one of the more challenging activities that most of us encounter in our everyday lives and requires significantly greater effort than walking uphill. Walking uphill requires significantly greater effort than walking on a flat surface and each of those activities requires significantly greater effort than sitting on the couch watching TV or sipping a martini; or sitting on the couch watching TV *and* sipping a martini (or sitting on a martini watching the couch).

In addition to the activity itself, we must also consider the conditions under which each activity takes place. Sticking with our stair-climbing example, most people find it much more taxing to walk up a flight of stairs on a hot, humid day or after indulging in a big meal as compared to when weather conditions are more favorable; or shortly after you've taken your rescue inhaler. In addition, various other factors can also negatively impact your breathing, such as anxiety, indoor and outdoor air pollution; or having a cold, flu, or pulmonary exacerbation, among many, many others. As I say over and over (and over) again, breathing is multi-factorial.

With this concept in mind, it can be helpful to observe the activities that cause you the most difficulty, as well as the related demands they put upon your respiratory, cardiovascular, muscular and skeletal systems...*and your emotional mind.* It is also helpful to understand that there are ways we can increase the supply side of the equation as well, using various strategies and techniques. The purpose of this chapter is to help you evaluate your own activities of daily living (ADL) and to understand how these various factors affect you, as well as what you can do to stack the odds in your favor.

Keep in mind that you won't always be able to change the physical requirements of an activity, and even more rarely will you be able to change the external environment. However, once you become attuned to which factors have the greatest impact on your performance, both positive and negative, you will be able to incorporate practices such as controlled breathing techniques, optimal timing of your medications, and using your supplemental oxygen to your greatest advantage; in addition to avoiding respiratory triggers such as pollution, temperature and weather extremes; and allergens.

Just because an activity makes you uncomfortable doesn't necessarily mean that it has to be avoided completely, and in many cases, quite the opposite is true. It shouldn't be. Remember that your body gets good at what you ask it (or don't ask it) to do, and over time, gradually increasing these difficult activities can actually *improve* your ability. However, in order to improve your performance, you will need to find ways to become more efficient and effective at performing these activities, so you can once again regain control of your breathing and your life; in other words, you will need to work smarter, not harder. Let's take a look at some of the factors that play a role in breathing and activity.

NOTE: As always, please clear any intended lifestyle changes with your physician.

Aerobic Capacity

Aerobic capacity refers to the efficiency and effectiveness with which your body utilizes oxygen to support physiologic activity. This is largely based on three main factors.

- How effectively your lungs move air in and out.
- How effectively your heart pumps blood.
- How efficiently your skeletal muscles utilize oxygen?

As I have mentioned previously, a problem in any one of these areas can impact your performance. However, if you have problems in more than one area, such as heart *and* lung disease, you will likely have significantly greater difficulty than either one alone.

Air Supply and Oxygen Demand: Respiratory Mechanics and Metabolism

In order for us to take a breath, the brain sends a signal down the spinal cord to the phrenic nerve, which innervates the diaphragm, activating it to contract downward. This downward contraction creates a negative pressure in the thoracic cavity, causing the lungs to fill with air. Various factors can either positively or negatively influence the effectiveness of this pressurized system. As an example, patients with emphysema can have increased thoracic pressures due to hyperinflation of the lungs. Similarly, pressure in the abdominal cavity can increase due to a large meal, gas, or constipation.

Increased pressure in either the thoracic or abdominal cavities can impair the diaphragm's ability to contract due to increased pressure pushing either down from above or up from below, respectively. Increased pressure in both cavities at the same time will impair breathing even further, as in the case of someone with hyper-inflated lungs who just ate a big meal; or simply bending over to tie your shoe, compressing both cavities.

People with obstructive lung diseases typically have difficulty with *exhalation*; i.e. moving air *out* and people with restrictive lung diseases typically have difficulty with *inhalation*; i.e. moving air *in*. However, inhalation and exhalation are like Yin and Yang, meaning that if you have difficulty with one phase, it will also affect the other, with the end result being the same; shortness of breath, decreased muscle strength and decreased activity tolerance. This explains why you can be short of breath even in the presence of normal or even high oxygen content in the blood, i.e. saturation.

In the case of a strictly mechanical problem, supplemental oxygen will not help you. Instead, the solution lies in performing the controlled breathing techniques, clearing your secretions, and taking your rescue inhaler, in the short term; and gradual, but progressive exercise, over the long term. That being said, respiratory mechanics *can* affect metabolism and oxygen saturation. In the case where your shortness of breath *is* accompanied by a decrease in oxygen saturation, you *will* benefit from supplemental oxygen, adjusting or *titrating* the amount based upon your pulse oximeter readings. In fact, if your oxygen saturation falls below 90%, I would *strongly* recommend speaking with your doctor about supplemental oxygen use.

Finally, on the flip side, there are a group of people who are hypoxic, yet do not feel particularly breathless. This often occurs in people who have been living with a respiratory disease for a long period of time as they have become desensitized to their dyspnea. In this situation, you should also be using supplemental oxygen, adjusting or *titrating* the amount based upon your oximeter readings. If your oxygen saturation is in the nineties, preferably 93% plus, you're good. If your saturation is below 90%, turn up the oxygen or switch from a cannula to a mask. This is what I mean when I talk about "relying on your instruments," as opposed to making adjustments based solely on how you are feeling at that particular moment.

Body Positioning

Many people with pulmonary conditions have a difficult time breathing in certain positions, particularly, bending over and/or lying flat. Think about these positions in the context of thoracic and abdominal expansion. Both of these extremes create maximal compression (either in flexion or extension) of both the thorax and abdomen, increasing the pressure against which, the diaphragm has to contract. This is the result of actual physical and mechanical constraints, which explains why activities such as bending over to tie your shoe or lying flat on your back are difficult for so many people.

Upper Body Activity and the Open Chain

People with pulmonary conditions can also find upper body activity to be particularly difficult. As we've previously discussed in the context of better breathing techniques and recovery from shortness of breath; open chain activities refer to activities during which, the arms are free to move around in space. This puts the diaphragm and other respiratory muscles of the back, chest, shoulders, and thorax at a mechanical disadvantage—particularly when the arms are overhead. In contrast, when you "close the chain"—as in the case of leaning forward on your elbows or holding on to a treadmill or walker—the muscles of your chest, back and shoulders work in their reverse action, aiding ribcage elevation and thoracic expansion. This explains why activities such as washing or brushing your hair, reaching for something on a high shelf; even brushing your teeth or shaving; can be difficult.

Energy Cost and Metabolic Equivalents

MET level or metabolic equivalents are a measurement of physiologic workload or exercise tolerance; in other words, the energy cost of the activity. Every activity comes with its own metabolic price tag, which corresponds to the amount of oxygen consumed. Activities that are less than three METs are considered light. Activities between three and six METs are considered moderate and activities that are six METs or greater are considered heavy or vigorous activity.

Below are some sample activities and their corresponding MET level. Please keep in mind that these are *rough* estimates and *many* factors can affect individual MET level.

- 1 MET: energy expenditure at rest, lying in bed
- 1.0 to 1.9 METs: eating, grooming, shaving (sitting), writing
- 2.0 to 2.9 METs: cooking, making the bed, showering (warm), dressing (sitting)
- 3.0 to 3.9 METs: vacuuming, showering (warm), dressing (standing), walk 3 mph
- 4.0 to 4.9 METs: gardening, swimming,
- 5.0 to 5.9 METs: Showering (hot, standing)
- 6.0 to 6.9 METs: stair climbing (down)

Activities of Daily Living

When I recently polled the members of my *Ultimate Pulmonary Wellness Facebook Group*, the three activities that were reported to be most difficult were stair climbing, walking uphill, and walking quickly…*by a landslide.* As I mentioned at the beginning of this chapter, walking up a flight of stairs requires significantly more effort than walking on an incline i.e. uphill; and walking uphill; sometimes even if it's only a slight incline; requires significantly more effort than walking on flat ground.

Walking

Like breathing itself, locomotion in all of its forms is a multi-factorial process that both *affects* and is *affected by* many variables. Walking increases your body's demand for both air (mechanical) and oxygen (metabolic). For that reason, it is important for us to have strategies at our disposal to either reduce the energy demands of the activity or to increase the supply of air and oxygen.

Other factors to consider include: the longer and steeper the stairs, the greater the metabolic demand. The faster you walk, the greater the demand. Carrying something while you walk, or walking and talking will also increase the demand; and just in case you're sensing a theme here, the more challenging the activity, the greater the demand. Emotional factors like anxiety can also play a role; both affecting and being affected by breathing and activity, decreasing the supply of air *and* increasing the metabolic demand.

Here are some techniques you can incorporate when you're walking:

Practice "the Breathing."

When it comes to walking, by far, the greatest tools you have to help reduce the demands of the activity and increase your supply of air and oxygen are your controlled breathing techniques. Diaphragmatic, pursed-lip and paced breathing will give you greater breath control, allowing you to walk more. Time your breathing with your walking, with each step being one count. Try breathing in for two steps and out for four steps or whichever pattern you find most beneficial. The same is true for stair climbing, using each step as a count of one. If this is too vigorous, you can modify the activity even further. Instead of one step for each count, breathe in while standing still and exhale as you start to climb again.

Pace Yourself!

Walk as slowly as you need to in order to maintain control of your breathing. Walking at a slower pace will reduce the metabolic demand of the activity. If you're still having trouble maintaining control of your breathing, stop walking and perform the techniques for *recovery from shortness of breath*. Once you have regained control of your breathing, you can start walking again…*slowly*.

Take your "rescue" medication before exercise or activity.

Taking your rescue medication; typically, a short-acting bronchodilator; increases the supply of air and oxygen by opening up the airways, allowing you to take a deeper breath. Taking it approximately 15 minutes before exercise should help you have your best workout.

Increase your supplemental oxygen as necessary.

If your oxygen saturation drops below 90%, increase the liter flow or switch to a mask.

Use a shopping cart or rolling walker.

Using a shopping cart or rolling walker closes the chain, improving respiratory mechanics; not only decreasing the metabolic demand of the activity, but also increasing the supply of air and oxygen.

Relax!!!

I realize that this is usually easier said than done. However, *try* to prepare yourself mentally and emotionally for the activity. As an example, before you start up a flight of stairs, take a moment or two to compose yourself and start your controlled breathing techniques proactively, *before* starting up the stairs.

Shhh...

Many people find walking and talking difficult. Talking is essentially continuous exhaling, which will quickly reduce your available supply of air. Pace your breathing so that you are speaking during what would normally be the exhalation phase, and by taking slow, deep breaths in between speaking, while the other person is talking. Think of it as an opportunity to work on your listening skills.

Lifting and Carrying

Lifting and carrying, especially heavy objects, can significantly impair your breathing from both a supply and demand perspective. First, lifting and carrying will increase the metabolic demand to varying degrees, depending upon the load. As the load increases, so will the metabolic demand. In addition, lifting and carrying can also decrease supply. Imagine carrying a paper bag of groceries across your chest in front of you. This compresses the thorax, mechanically preventing you from taking a deep breath.

Now think about carrying two plastic bags, one in each hand. This load pulls down on the thorax and the ribcage, increasing the amount of resistance required by the diaphragm to elevate the ribcage, again, preventing you from taking a deep breath. Again, the same factors including walking on a flat surface, walking on an incline, and climbing stairs, will further increase the metabolic requirements.

Bending and Reaching

Bending and reaching compress your thoracic and abdominal cavities like an accordion, increasing the pressures against which, the diaphragm has to contract, preventing you from taking a deep breath. There is further compression of the thorax, preventing you from taking a deep breath and preventing the lungs from filling with air.

Another task people regularly report difficulty with is bending down to tie their shoes. This is due to thoracic and abdominal compression. Instead of trying to breathe while you are down there, prepare yourself by taking a deep breath in before you bend and slowly and gently exhale through pursed lips as you bend down and tie your shoe. As you start to run short on air, rise up again as you take a deep inhalation. Then exhale through pursed lips as you bend over to tie the other shoe.

Showering and Bathing

Many people find showering and bathing extremely difficult. For both of these activities, there are *many* factors—almost like an "all of the above" situation. Increased humidity in the bathroom due to the hot water and steam can make you work harder to move air in *and* out. Think of inhaling and exhaling that thick air as being similar to drinking a milkshake through a narrow straw as compared to plain water. Instead of hot, use lukewarm or tepid water and leave the bathroom door either cracked or completely open.

Another issue has to do with the use of the upper extremities to wash; especially overhead as you do when you wash your hair. As we have discussed many times, this open chain activity puts the diaphragm and the respiratory muscles at a very poor mechanical advantage, significantly increasing your shortness of breath. In order to decrease the work of breathing as well as the overall metabolic demand of showering, I would suggest using a shower chair or bench, as well as a hand-held shower. This will allow you to relax and focus on your breathing as you sit and wash your body, as opposed to constantly worrying about shortness of breath or worse, slipping and falling. And while we're on the subject, let me tell you that those hand-held showers are *delightful.*

Finally, if you have oxygen, turn it up if you need to. Now, just so there are no misunderstandings, showering or bathing is a situation in which you simply *cannot* "rely on your instruments." So please *do not* take your pulse oximeter into the shower with you or you will have a whole different set of problems to deal with (or maybe you won't). Also, if you prefer to take a bath instead of a shower, *please* be careful. Make sure that you are able to lower yourself into and lift yourself out of the tub *safely.*

Dressing

Getting dressed goes hand in hand with bathing. For many of the same reasons that bathing is difficult, drying yourself off and dressing can be equally, if not more difficult. Again, overhead, open chain movements like toweling dry or putting on a shirt put the diaphragm at a mechanical disadvantage. To overcome this difficulty, try putting on a terrycloth bathrobe to do the drying for you, while you sit and catch your breath.

As you are getting dressed, use your controlled breathing techniques, coordinating movement with exhalation and inhaling in between. As an example, inhale for a count of two. Exhale for a count of four as you put one arm in the sleeve. Inhale for a count of two. Exhale as you put your other arm in the other sleeve. The same principles apply to pants, socks, shoes, etc.

Cleaning and Housework

Chores like laundry (bending, lifting, carrying, reaching); vacuuming (bending, pushing, pulling, reaching); and making the bed (bending, pulling, reaching), are also difficult for people with respiratory problems due to the increased physical and metabolic demands, positioning, and many other challenges. Add to these issues, the potential for exposure to unhealthy environmental and chemical triggers that can add insult (and inflammation) to injury. Tasks like dusting, vacuuming, sweeping, mopping, etcetera, etcetera expose us to all kinds of potential bacteria, viruses, allergens, and other respiratory triggers in the form of dust, debris, mold, insects and animals, and their excrement; as well as the cleaning supplies themselves, among others. Any of these factors can quickly trigger the inflammatory response, constricting the airways and increasing the production of mucus, and the work of breathing. They can also make us sick. If in doubt, please don't do it yourself. At a minimum, wear a mask, ventilate the room, use an air purifier and please choose your cleaning products carefully, opting for hypo- or ideally, non-allergenic.

Sexual Activity

Although not often talked about, sex is also a big concern for many patients. Sexual activity involves an increased mechanical and metabolic demand for air, oxygen, circulation, and aerobic capacity due to the elevated workload. In addition, there are also complex emotional aspects that can contribute to the situation, for better and for worse. Sex can be a wonderful and enjoyable experience for many people, or an extremely anxiety-provoking situation for many others—especially if you are concerned about being able to breathe, in addition to enjoying yourself and pleasing your partner.

As with other activities, a little preparation beforehand will go a long way. Think about which positions will allow you to breathe more easily while decreasing the physical and emotional demands of the activity. As an example, lying on your back may decrease your demand for air and oxygen, reducing the aerobic requirements of the activity. However, you may also need to consider how your breathing will be affected by the weight of your partner. In that case, you may want to try other positions. If you need oxygen, turn it up! If you have a rescue inhaler, ask your doctor if you can use it proactively.

Now, while I'm not trying to give you the *Kama Sutra for Pulmonary Patients*, my suggestion would be for you and your partner to experiment with various positions and practices to figure out what works best *for both of you*. Although it may be uncomfortable at first, communication is key to finding strategies that meet both partners' needs. And *breathe*! Utilize all of the controlled breathing techniques, before, during, and after sex. Just be sure to skip the requisite after–sex cigarette.

Energy Conservation versus Energy Maximization

At first glance, the difference between energy conservation and energy maximization seem like nitpicking or semantics. However, there are significant differences between the two ideas; with *mindset* often being a *major* factor. In my experience, "traditional" energy conservation techniques typically focus on teaching people how to modify the activity in a downward direction to accommodate the metabolic demand. Paradoxically, while this downgrade may make the activity more manageable for the moment, it will ultimately make it become more difficult over time. Remember that your body gets good at doing what you ask it to do.

Finally, while I concede that there will be times that your limitations may get the best of you, I would much rather you take the steps to up your game to meet this increased demand as opposed to automatically downgrading all of your activities. I assure you that I am *not* minimizing your struggle. I *am* encouraging you *not* to sell the farm too quickly. My goal is to encourage you to keep trying, even when things get tough. Perhaps you need to work smarter, not harder.

CHAPTER 5

ULTIMATE PULMONARY WELLNESS

***"The whole is greater than the sum of its parts."* – Aristotle**

In today's healthcare environment, an overwhelming percentage of resources are spent on treating diseases and their associated manifestations. While treatment of disease is an essential part of wellness, there is far more to being healthy than simply not being sick. Instead of merely trying to eliminate illness, true *wellness* is the goal we are striving for—and can be achieved through a combination of positive life changes, education, and enlightenment, all of which can have a potentially powerful impact on both disease treatment and *prevention.*

With that in mind, my goal is to present you with the information that I have found to be the *most* successful and *most* practical over the past 25 years as well as to help guide you in determining which ones will work and which ones won't work *for you.*

If you read the classic literature on pulmonary rehabilitation, you will find hundreds of articles stating that after participation in a pulmonary rehabilitation program, participants feel better, can do more, and are less short of breath. However, most of these same articles will also state that pulmonary rehabilitation *does not* improve pulmonary function, which can often be disappointing for people.

Even though we do not necessarily agree with these findings, what this tells us is that if you feel better, can do more, and are less short of breath, without any improvement in pulmonary function, there have to be other factors involved in how well or how poorly you breathe—things like fitness level, nutrition, and emotional state. This is great news because these are things that we actually have some control over.

In this chapter, we will set the stage for the next several months, years, and hopefully the rest of your life, by identifying the *most* important principles of Ultimate Pulmonary Wellness.

Let's start with a few definitions:

Ultimate: The dictionary defines "ultimate" as consummate, maximum, most, or to the highest degree or quantity. Sounds impressive, right? I would also add "quality" to this description because I hear people say over and over again—and I also believe—that *quality* of life is equally if not more important than quantity. Our goal is not just for you to feel pretty good. Our goal is for you to feel *amazing* and to achieve the absolute maximal level of health, function, and quality of life possible.

Pulmonary: "Pulmonary" pertains to the lungs and the respiratory system. When I ask people to rate their understanding of their condition or even the basics of the respiratory system, most people report around a C+ grade level. I don't know about you but if you're living with a chronic pulmonary disease and you have only a C+ understanding of the respiratory system, I consider this a problem.

In an ideal world, when you receive a diagnosis like Chronic Obstructive Pulmonary Disease (COPD), Idiopathic Pulmonary Fibrosis (IPF), Pulmonary Hypertension (PH), or any other serious medical condition, it would be wonderful if you could spend an hour or two with your doctor, asking questions and taking notes about all the things that you will need to know.

However, in today's fast-paced healthcare environment, doctors are often so busy that even the greatest, most caring physicians simply do not have the time to teach you everything that you need to know about your illness. That's my other motivation for writing this book.

Wellness: Often, when we seek medical care, we are focused on the exact opposite of wellness. In fact, as a society, we spend far more resources battling sickness than promoting true wellness. Typically, when patients first report their symptoms to their doctor (shortness of breath, cough, or the inability to walk uphill), the first treatments will almost always be medication (or more likely, medications).

However, not enough thought is given to the other factors that come into play when it comes to breathing. Lifestyle choices can either make you feel better or worse depending on which ones you choose to do—or not do—things like exercise, eating a healthier diet, quitting smoking, taking steps to manage stress and anxiety, and *prevention* of infection.

The Formula

Ultimate Pulmonary Wellness can be divided into five major categories, with each one accounting for *approximately* 20% of total pulmonary and overall health. Those 5 categories are Medical, Exercise, Nutrition, Management of Stress and Anxiety, and Prevention of Infection.

I will touch on these areas briefly in this chapter in order to give you an overview of the program and to highlight the role of each of these components in your health and wellbeing. Later in the book, there will be a chapter for each topic that goes into much greater detail and gives you specific guidelines and suggestions for each.

Medical (20%)

To me, good medicine means having the right doctor or doctors, taking the right medications and taking those medications properly. People ask me all the time "How do you know if you have the right doctor?" At the most basic level, you probably want a doctor who is smart, experienced, and compassionate. After that, most of us look for any variety of other qualities and character traits. What characteristics do you look for in a doctor? We will help you clarify some of your own physician "makes" or "breaks."

When it comes to medications, taking the proper medicines is heavily dependent upon having the right doctor but getting the most benefit from your medicines also depends upon taking them at the right times and in the correct order, as well as using the delivery devices properly. We will discuss these topics in greater detail later in the book, as this is an area that I particularly hope to make crystal clear.

Exercise (20%)

When we discussed shortness of breath, we talked about the fact that people often avoid activities that cause them shortness of breath. Consequently, all of the muscles that you use to do those activities get weaker and your body becomes less efficient at using oxygen. In addition to teaching you specific breathing exercises, I will guide you through the most beneficial exercises and help you put together a program that will be most effective and best suited *for you*.

Nutrition (20%)

When it comes to nutrition, in addition to eating a balanced and healthy diet, there are certain concepts that relate particularly to pulmonary disease. These include topics like mechanics of eating and breathing or being at your correct (healthy) weight. In addition, there are certain foods that will help you fight your disease and its associated symptoms, while others will make them worse.

Stress and Anxiety Management/Meditation (20%)

Anxiety and depression can have a devastating impact on someone living with a pulmonary disease. To make matters worse, living with a pulmonary disease can cause a tremendous amount of anxiety and depression. This is another cycle that we hope to break so that you can be less stressed and live a happier, healthier, more satisfying life.

Prevention of Infection (20%)

The final piece of the puzzle is prevention of infection. To be clear, a cold or infection for someone with a respiratory disease can be far more serious than for someone who is otherwise healthy. Plus, people with lung disease often don't get a little infection. They get big infections and their infections often go right to the chest.

Because the respiratory system is your weak link, it is crucial that you implement some type of *prevention* strategy. This effort will be well worth your while, as it is often easier to prevent an infection than to treat one once you've got it. I will give you a number of tools and suggestions to help you in your fight against infection.

Everything Else (10-100%)

Since we believe in giving 110%, there is an additional 10% left over for a category I like to call "everything else." What I mean by "everything else" is that even if you do everything right including the "*big five*" of pulmonary wellness, there will always be factors outside of our control. Being superstitious by nature, I don't want to name any of them here but take a deep breath, keep living your life, and expect the unexpected.

How to Use This Book

Now, let's take each of these "big five" one at a time and expand upon them in a way that will give you a very clear and comprehensive understanding of what factors will help you live a better life and which ones might make your life more difficult. This book is organized so you can go chapter by chapter or you can choose to skip around. So, please, make yourself comfortable and feel free to use the information in whatever fashion makes the most sense to you.

CHAPTER 6
MEDICATIONS

"Drugs don't work if patients don't take them (properly)."
– Former US Surgeon General, C. Everett Koop, MD

Written with gratitude to my Co-Author, Mark Mangus, Sr., BSRC, RRT, RPFT, FAARC

When it comes to living well with a pulmonary disease, fewer topics are less clearly understood than how to take your medications most effectively in order to get the maximum benefit from their use. If you have any doubts about this, just go to any online pulmonary support group and type in "how…" or "in what order should I take my medications." I can assure you that within a few minutes, you will receive a virtual plethora of responses, comments, instructions and opinions. Some of them may come from lay-people—patients and caregivers, some may come from clinicians and other professional people, and some of them *may* even be correct. Unfortunately, many others will be based on misinformation, misunderstanding, misconception, myth or urban legend.

There are several reasons why this is so. First, the information, itself, is complex and in many cases, counterintuitive. The names of the medications seem to be in another language and their delivery devices can often be difficult to use. In addition, most (or at least, many) clinicians spend far too little time (if any) teaching their patients about their medications and making sure that they understand how to use them properly. It also doesn't help that there is often disagreement, even among clinicians as to what works best. When you add all of these things up, is it really any wonder patients are confused?

For this important chapter, I have asked my friend and colleague, Mark Mangus, Sr., BSRC, RRT, RPFT, FAARC, (or as I like to call him, *Respiratory Therapist-Laureate*), to be my co-author. Mr. Mangus and I have been wrangling with people (and each other) for years over this important topic and for this chapter, in particular, we really wanted to get it right; so we can provide you with the absolute best and most current information, in a way that is also easy to understand and put into use.

Throughout this chapter, Mr. Mangus and I hope to clarify many important aspects of medication use and to suggest ways that will help you derive the most benefit from your own program. We will be presenting our best observations—information that we have gathered over the past 25 years working in cardiopulmonary physical therapy and rehabilitation; and EMS for me; and more than 40 years working in virtually every aspect of respiratory care for Mark.

DISCLAIMER: Please understand that we are *not* telling you what you should or shouldn't do. *Please…do not* alter your routine because "Noah and Mark told me to." That is *not* what we are doing. One more time: *do not* make *any* changes to your medication regimen based upon our observations without first discussing them with your physician and getting his or her okay.

Before getting into any of the actual medications, I think it would be helpful to provide you with a short glossary of terms so that if you do get lost, you will have a quick reference guide to help you get back on track. Once you understand these definitions, knowing which medication you take, why you take it, and how you should take it, should make much more sense.

Bronchoconstriction, Bronchodilation, and Inflammation

The prefix, "broncho" means relating to the bronchi or airways. As we have previously discussed, the airways begin with the trachea or windpipe, which first splits into the right and left mainstem bronchi. These airways continue to branch into smaller and smaller bronchi, bronchioles and alveoli, the tiny air sacs where gas exchange occurs.

Bronchoconstriction is the constriction, narrowing, or contraction of the smooth muscle lining the airways (bronchi and bronchioles).

Bronchodilation is the dilation, widening, or relaxation of the smooth muscle lining the airways (bronchi and bronchioles).

Inflammation is the body's response to harmful stimuli or alien invaders. In the airways, inflammation causes swelling of the smooth muscle lining the inside of the airways and an increase in mucus production.

Bronchoconstriction, bronchodilation and inflammation all have their place in the normal functioning of a healthy respiratory system. As an example, imagine you're walking outside on a hot summer day. Suddenly, a bus drives past you, spewing soot and who knows what else from its exhaust, right in your face. In response, your airways constrict and mucus production increases in order to protect you by trapping that airborne junk before it has a chance to enter your lower respiratory tract and lungs.

The problem arises, however, when inflammation, bronchoconstriction and increased mucus production become excessive or a more chronic, or permanent state as opposed to just a normal, healthy response to a trigger or alien invader.

Agonist versus Antagonist

An *agonist* is a chemical that binds to a specific receptor, causing a biological or physiological response. In other words, an agonist has a positive, pro- or stimulatory effect, increasing the action of those receptors.

An *antagonist* is the opposite of an agonist. An antagonist works by blocking or reducing a biological or physiological response. In other words, it has a negative, anti- or inhibitory effect, *decreasing* the action of those receptors.

Taking Your Medication Correctly: Easy as ABC!

This may sound crazy, but I have been trying to figure out an easy way for patients to keep their medications straight for years...*literally*!!! One day, it finally came to me in a song: ABC! 123! OMG! How could I have not seen this...*for years*??? As the Jackson 5 told us: "ABC, it's easy as one, two, three, Baby, you and me!" Now, you may be wondering what this song has to do with pulmonary medications. That's a good question and here is a good answer.

Inhaled pulmonary medications generally fall into one of two general categories, Bronchodilators and Corticosteroids. As the name implies, bronchodilators open up or *dilate* the airways. Corticosteroids reduce inflammation and edema (swelling) in the airways. Bronchodilators can be further broken down into two classes: Anticholinergics (now often referred to as Anti-Muscarinics or Muscarinic Antagonists) and Beta-2 Adrenergic Receptor Agonists or Beta-2 Agonists.

NOTE: For the purposes of this chapter (and ease of understanding), we will use the term anticholinergics as opposed to anti-muscarinic or muscarinic antagonist.

So...

A=Anticholinergic

B=Beta-2 Agonist

C=Corticosteroid (Inhaled)

Often, people with respiratory disease are prescribed one medication from each of the 3 classes, A, B, and C—in other words, one anticholinergic (A), one beta-2 agonist (B) and one corticosteroid (C). It reminds me of the old-style Chinese restaurant menus: one from Column A, one from Column B and one from Column C. These can be prescribed either as separate medications or as one of the combination medications now available. Many people are also prescribed a rescue inhaler for emergency use; typically, a short-acting beta-2 agonist to be taken either at regularly scheduled intervals or PRN (i.e. "as needed").

There are certain things that you will need to understand if you want to get the maximum benefit from your medications. Remember, our goal is to maximally increase bronchodilation, decrease bronchoconstriction and reduce or prevent inflammation, all for as long as possible.

In order to achieve these goals, it is important to understand what medication(s) you take, why you take them, when you should take them and how you should take them. If you haven't figured it out by now, you are the "who."

Medication Class: *Learning Your ABC's*

Anticholinergics (A)

The *parasympathetic nervous system* can be thought of as the "*rest and digest*" division of the autonomic nervous system. Its activity is primarily mediated by the neurotransmitter, *acetylcholine*. The *cholinergic* action of the parasympathetic nervous system on the lungs and the respiratory system, particularly on the *muscarinic* acetylcholine receptors causes bronchoconstriction.

BOTTOM LINE: Anticholinergics block or reduce bronchoconstriction, which, as Martha Stewart might say, "is a good thing."

Table 1: Anticholinergics (A)

Generic Name	Brand Name
ipratropium bromide	**ATROVENT**
aclidinium bromide	**TUDORZA**
tiotropium bromide	**SPIRIVA**
umeclidinium bromide	**INCRUSE ELLIPTA**
glycopyrrolate bromide	**SEEBRI NEOHALER**

*Shaded areas indicate long-acting drugs.

Beta-2 Adrenergic Receptor Agonists or Beta-2 Agonists (B)

The *sympathetic nervous system* can be thought of as the "fight or flight" division of the autonomic nervous system. Its activity is primarily mediated by the neurotransmitter, *adrenaline* or *epinephrine*. The *adrenergic* action of the sympathetic nervous system on the lungs and the respiratory system, particularly on the beta-2 adrenergic receptors causes bronchodilation.

BOTTOM LINE: Beta-2 agonists stimulate or increase bronchodilation, which again, as Martha Stewart might say, "is also a good thing."

Table 2: Beta-2 Agonists (B)

Generic	Brand Name
albuterol sulfate	**PROAIR, VENTOLIN, PROVENTIL**
levalbuterol tartrate	**XOPENEX**
terbutaline	**BRETHAIRE**
salmeterol xinafoate	**SEREVENT**
formoterol fumarate	**FORADIL, PERFOROMIST**
aformoterol tartrate	**BROVANA**
indacaterol	**ARCAPTA NEOHALER**
indacaterol maleate	**ONBREZ BREEZHALER**
olodaterol	**STRIVERDI RESPIMAT**

*Shaded areas indicate long-acting drugs.

Short-Acting versus Long-Acting versus Ultra-Long-Acting

Both anticholinergics and beta-2 agonists are available in short-acting, long-acting, and ultra-long-acting formulations. As we talk about pulmonary medications, you will often hear terms like SAMA, SABA, LAMA, and LABA. Every once in a while, you may hear a "Rama Lama Ding Dong" thrown in for good measure. These abbreviations refer to two things: duration or how long they last (short-acting versus long-acting) and the class of medication.

SA=Short-Acting. Short-acting medications have a rapid onset of action (1-5 minutes) and typically achieve their peak effect within 15-20 minutes. Their effects typically last up to 4-6 hours.

SAMA=Short-Acting Muscarinic Antagonist (anticholinergic)

SABA=Short-Acting Beta-2 Agonist

Due to their rapid onset of action, short-acting bronchodilators are often referred to as "rescue medications". These are the medications that you should carry around with you and take when you need quick relief.

LA=Long-Acting. Long-acting medications have a slower onset of action with their effects lasting up to 12 hours. For this reason, they are usually taken twice per day (every 12 hours).

LAMA=Long-Acting Muscarinic Antagonist (anticholinergic)

LABA=Long-Acting Beta-2 Agonist

Ultra-Long-Acting medications can last for up to 24 hours. For this reason, they are usually taken once per day (every 24 hours).

Due to their long duration of effectiveness, long-acting and ultra-long-acting bronchodilators are often referred to as "maintenance" or "preventer" medications, although my personal preference is to reserve the terms "maintenance" and "preventer" for the anti-inflammatories.

IMPORTANT: Long-Acting and Ultra-Long-Acting Bronchodilators should NOT be taken in an emergency due to their longer onset of action.

Corticosteroids (C)

Corticosteroids, also known simply as "steroids" or anti-inflammatories reduce inflammation and edema (swelling) in the airways. They work on a long-term basis and are often referred to as "preventer medications" since their goal is to reduce and ideally, prevent inflammation before it occurs. These medications work over the long-term, meaning that unlike bronchodilators, there is no immediate impact on airway activity. Therefore, you should not expect to feel any different right after you take it. In fact, corticosteroids can often take days or even weeks to achieve their peak effect.

BOTTOM LINE: Corticosteroids reduce inflammation.

Table 3: Corticosteroids (C)

Generic	Brand Name
beclomethasone dipropionate	QVAR
budesonide	PULMICORT
ciclesonide	ALVESCO
flunisolide	AEROBID
fluticasone	FLOVENT
mometasone	ASMANEX
triamcinolone acetoide	AZMACORT
fluticasone furoate	ARNUITY ELLIPTA

IMPORTANT: Unlike bronchodilators, corticosteroids *do not* directly dilate the airways. For that reason, corticosteroids should *never* be taken as a rescue medication.

NOTE: Corticosteroids often have a bad reputation because of their many side effects, which can include weight gain, osteoporosis, thinning of the skin, elevated blood sugar and ease of bruising. However, as compared to *oral* or *intravenous (IV)* medications, *inhaled* corticosteroids go directly to the respiratory system, with minimal amounts entering the systemic circulation. As a result, inhaled corticosteroids have significantly less side effects as their oral or IV counterparts.

COMBINATION MEDICATIONS

In recent years, a number of products have been approved that combine 2 classes of medication in one delivery device.

Table 4: Short-Acting Anticholinergic and Short-Acting Beta-2 Agonist

The first combination medications to become available contain ipratropium bromide, a short-acting anticholinergic, and albuterol sulfate, a short-acting beta-2 agonist.

BRAND NAME	Anticholinergic	Beta-2 Agonist
COMBIVENT (MDI)	ipratropium bromide	albuterol sulfate
DUONEB (nebulizer)	ipratropium bromide	albuterol sulfate

Table 5: Long-Acting Beta-2 Agonist and Inhaled Corticosteroid

The next combination medications to become available contain a long-acting beta-2 agonist and an inhaled corticosteroid.

BRAND NAME	Beta-2 Agonists	Corticosteroid
ADVAIR	salmeterol	fluticasone propionate
SYMBICORT	formoterol fumarate dihydrate	budesonide
DULERA	formoterol fumarate dihydrate	mometasone furoate
BREO ELLIPTA	vilanterol	fluticasone furoate

IMPORTANT: Long-Acting combination medications should *not* be taken in an emergency due to their longer time to onset of action.

Table 6: Long-Acting Anticholinergics and Long-Acting Beta-2 Agonist

Most recently, both long-acting and ultra-long-acting anticholinergic/ beta-2 agonist (dual bronchodilator) combinations have become available.

BRAND NAME	Anticholinergic	Beta-2 Agonist
BEVESPI AEROSPHERE	glycopyrrolate	formoterol fumarate
ANORO ELLIPTA	umeclidinium	vilanterol
ULTIBRO BREEZEHALER	glycopyrronium bromide	indacaterol maleate
ULTIBRON NEOHALER	glycopyrrolate	indacaterol
STIOLTO RESPIMAT	tiotropium bromide	olodaterol

IMPORTANT: Long-Acting combination medications should *not* be taken in an emergency due to their longer time to onset of action.

Use the chart below to identify *your* medications.

Bronchodilators				Inhaled	
Anticholinergics		**B**eta-2 Agonists		**C**orticosteroids	
Generic	**Brand**	**Generic**	**Brand**	**Generic**	**Brand**
ipratropium bromide	**ATROVENT**	albuterol sulfate	**PROVENTIL, VENTOLIN, PROAIR**	beclomethasone dipropionate	**QVAR**
tiotropium bromide	**SPIRIVA**	levalbuterol tartrate	**XOPENEX**	budesonide	**PULMICORT**
aclidinium bromide	**TUDORZA**	terbutaline	NONE	ciclesonide	**ALVESCO**
umeclidinium	**INCRUSE ELLIPTA**	salmeterol xinafoate	**SEREVENT**	flunisolide	**AEROBID**
glycopyrollate	**SEEBRI BREEZEHALER**	aformoterol tartrate	**BROVANA**	fluticasone	**FLOVENT**
		formoterol fumarate	**FORADIL, PERFOROMIST**	mometasone	**ASMANEX**
		indacaterol	**ARCAPTA NEOHALER**	triamcinolone acetoide	**AZMACORT**
		indacaterol maleate	**ONBREZ BREEZHALER**	fluticasone furoate	**ARNUITY ELLIPTA**
		oldaterol	**STRIVERDI RESPIMAT**		

*Shaded Areas Indicate Long-Acting Medications. **BOLD ALL CAPS Indicate Brand Names

(Updated April 18, 2017 by Noah Greenspan, DPT, CCS, EMT-B)

COMBINATION MEDICATIONS			
Brand Name	Bronchodilators		Inhaled
	Anticholinergics	**B**eta-2 Agonists	**C**orticosteroids
COMBIVENT, DUONEB	ipratropium bromide	albuterol	
ADVAIR		salmeterol	fluticasone propionate
SYMBICORT		formoterol fumarate dihydrate	budesonide
DULERA		formoterol fumarate dihydrate	mometasone furoate
BREO ELLIPTA		vilanterol	fluticasone furoate
ANORO ELLIPTA	umeclidinium	Vilanterol	
ULTIBRO BREEZEHALER	glycopyrronium bromide	indacaterol maleate	
ULTIBRON NEOHALER	glycopyrrolate	indacaterol	
STIOLTO RESPIMAT	tiotropium bromide	olodaterol	
BEVESPI AEROSPHERE	glycopyrrolate	formoterol fumarate	

*Shaded Areas Indicate Long-Acting Medications. **BOLD ALL CAPS Indicate Brand Names

(Updated April 18, 2017 by Noah Greenspan, DPT, CCS, EMT-B)

Timing is everything!

In addition to knowing what medications you take, it is also important to know when they should be taken. This applies to the specific order (if any) as well as properly spacing them out over the course of the day so that you get maximum effectiveness for the longest period of time.

While it would be impossible to address every person's individual medication regimen, we will explain the major principles and give you some *general* examples. However, questions concerning your own specific regimen should be addressed with your physician.

Let's assume that you are probably taking one (long-acting) medication from each class (anticholinergic, beta-2 agonist and corticosteroid) *plus* a rescue medication. These can either be taken individually or as part of a combination medication (combination 1 or combination 2).

3 Individual Medications: A + B + C

Anticholinergic + Beta-2 Agonist + Corticosteroid

Example: Spiriva (A) + Serevent (B) + Flovent (C)

If you are taking 3 separate medications, we would suggest taking the long-acting anticholinergic (A) first, followed by the long-acting beta-2 agonist (B) about 5-15 minutes later and finally, the Corticosteroid about 5-15 minutes after that.

RATIONALE: By separating these medications by 5-15 minutes each, the first bronchodilator (the anticholinergic) starts to work, allowing better delivery of the second bronchodilator (the beta-2 agonist). Then, both bronchodilators work together, allowing for the best delivery of the corticosteroid.

There is very good evidence suggesting that by taking the anticholinergic and beta-2 agonist in close proximity to each other, their effects are multiplied as compared to taking either one alone or further apart.

IMPORTANT: Immediately after you take the steroid, it is crucial that you rinse your mouth out, gargle, spit and repeat. The reason for this is that if the steroid remains in your mouth or throat, it can cause a fungal infection called thrush (oral candidiasis). This is another reason why taking the steroid last "is a good thing."

Combination 1: AB + C

Anticholinergic/Beta-2 Agonist Combination + Corticosteroid

Example: Anoro Ellipta (AB) + Pulmicort (C)

If you are taking a long-acting anticholinergic/beta-2 agonist combination *plus* a corticosteroid, we would suggest taking the anticholinergic/beta-2 agonist (AB) first, followed by the corticosteroid (C) about 5-15 minutes later.

RATIONALE: By separating these medications by 5-15 minutes, the anticholinergic/beta-2 agonist (both bronchodilators) start to work, allowing for better delivery of the corticosteroid.

IMPORTANT: Immediately after you take the steroid, it is crucial that you rinse your mouth, gargle, spit and repeat. The reason for this is that if the steroid remains in your mouth or throat, it can cause a fungal infection called thrush (oral candidiasis). This is another reason why taking the steroid last "is a good thing."

Combination 2: A + BC

Anticholinergic + Beta-2 Agonist/Corticosteroid Combination

Example: Spiriva (A) + Advair (BC)

If you are taking a long-acting anticholinergic *plus* a long-acting beta-2 agonist/corticosteroid combination, we would suggest taking the anticholinergic (A) first, followed by the beta-2 agonist/corticosteroid (BC) about 5-15 minutes later.

RATIONALE: By separating them by 5-15 minutes, the anticholinergic (bronchodilator) starts to work, allowing for better delivery of the beta-2 agonist and the corticosteroid.

IMPORTANT: Immediately after you take the steroid, it is crucial that you rinse your mouth, gargle, spit and repeat. The reason for this is that if the steroid remains in your mouth or throat, it can cause a fungal infection called thrush (oral candidiasis). This is another reason why taking the steroid last "is a good thing."

In each of these examples, the corticosteroid is *always* taken last. This is because it is the corticosteroid that will have the greatest *long-term* impact on reducing airway inflammation. For that reason, you want to take the steroid when your lungs are the most open (following maximal dilation), giving the medication the greatest chance of reaching the deeper areas of the airways (i.e. bronchi and bronchioles).

IMPORTANT: Once daily ultra-long-acting medications should be taken at the same time every day, 24 hours apart, so if you take it at 8 AM today, you should take it again at 8 AM tomorrow (and the next day and the next day). Remember, your body likes consistency.

Although some people think that *when* you take a once-daily medication doesn't matter (since it is once daily, anyway), we would suggest taking it in the morning. In this way, the medication's peak effect occurs during the day when you are likely to be the most active. In keeping with our principle of supply and demand, we want to have the greatest supply of air available to us when the demand for oxygen is greatest, which for most people is during the day.

Twice daily long-acting medications should also be taken at the same time every day, 12 hours apart. That means that if your first dose is at 8 AM, your second dose should be at 8 PM. Again, try to be as consistent as possible, remembering that your body likes consistency.

To put this concept in better perspective, let's say that you were to incorrectly take your long-acting medication at 8 AM and again at 6 PM. This is only 10 hours apart, which is too short. More importantly, this means that it will be 14 hours until your next dose, which is too long. Again, consistency is key!

Your 24-Hour Medication Plan

We have already discussed the order in which you should take your medications within each individual sitting. Now, let's put all of these pieces together in the context of your overall lifestyle and your activity level over the course of the day. Use the worksheets on the next pages to help you map out your most effective 24-hour medication schedule, timing your medications to both maximize their effectiveness and pair them with the appropriate level of activity.

As mentioned previously, you will make your long-acting medications the anchors around which you will build your overall schedule.

Let's go back to our previous examples.

3 Individual Medications: A + B + C

Anticholinergic + Beta-2 Agonist + Corticosteroid

Example: Spiriva (A) + Serevent (B) + Flovent (C)

If you are taking 3 separate medications (a long-acting anticholinergic or muscarinic antagonist + a long-acting beta-2 agonist + a corticosteroid), you could take all 3 medications at 8 AM. Since most long-acting anticholinergics (Spiriva and Tudorza) are only once-a-day medications, at 8 PM, you would only take the long-acting beta-2 Agonist + the corticosteroid. In between, you could fill in with your rescue medication, as prescribed by your doctor.

If you generally need your rescue medication, (e.g. albuterol), only once per day, you could try taking it at 2 PM, allowing for even spacing between your morning and evening doses of the long-acting medications. So, your schedule would look like this:

8 AM Spiriva + Serevent + Flovent

2 PM albuterol

8 PM Serevent + Flovent

If you generally need your rescue medication twice per day, you could try taking it at 12 noon and 4 PM, again, allowing for even spacing between your morning and evening doses of the long-acting medications.

So, your schedule would look like this:

8 AM Spiriva + Serevent + Flovent

12 Noon albuterol

4 PM albuterol

8 PM Serevent + Flovent

Combination 1: (A and B in combination) + C

Anticholinergic/Beta-2 Agonist Combination + Corticosteroid

Example: Anoro Ellipta (AB) + Pulmicort (C)

If you are taking a long-acting anticholinergic or muscarinic antagonist (LAMA)/long-acting beta-2 agonist combination, + a corticosteroid, you could take both medications at 8 AM. Since most long-acting anticholinergics/beta-2 agonist combination medications are only taken once daily, at 8 PM, you would only take the Corticosteroid. In between, you could fill in with your rescue medication, as prescribed by your doctor.

If you generally need your rescue medication, (e.g. albuterol), once per day, you could take it at 2 PM, allowing for even spacing between your morning and evening doses of the long-acting medications. So, your schedule would look like this:

8 AM Anoro Ellipta + Pulmicort

2 PM albuterol

8 PM Pulmicort

If you generally need your rescue medication twice per day, you could take it at 12 noon and 4 PM, allowing for even spacing between your morning and evening doses of the long-acting medications.

So, your schedule would look like this:

8 AM Anoro Ellipta + Pulmicort

12 Noon Albuterol

4 PM Albuterol

8 PM Pulmicort

Combination 2: A + (B and C in combination)

Anticholinergic + Beta-2 Agonist/Corticosteroid Combination

Spiriva (A) + Advair (BC)

If you are taking a long-acting anticholinergic or muscarinic antagonist (LAMA) + a long-acting beta-2 agonist/corticosteroid combination, you could take both medications at 8 AM. Since most long-acting anticholinergics (Spiriva and Tudorza) are once-daily medications, at 8 PM, you would only take the combination medication. In between, you could fill in with your rescue medication, as prescribed by your doctor.

If you generally need your rescue medication, (e.g. albuterol), once per day, you could take it at 2 PM, allowing for even spacing between your morning and evening doses of the long-acting medications. So, your schedule would look like this:

8 AM Spiriva + Advair

2 PM Albuterol

8 PM Advair

If you generally need your rescue medication twice per day, you could take it at 12 noon and 4 PM, allowing for even spacing between your morning and evening doses of the long-acting medications.

So, your schedule would look like this:

8 AM Spiriva + Advair

12 Noon Albuterol

4 PM Albuterol

8 PM Advair

How to Use Your Rescue Medication to Your Best Advantage

For many people, long-acting medications are sufficient to keep them breathing well all day. However, some individuals get tremendous benefit from the use of their short-acting (rescue) medication as a "booster". This can either be done at a regularly scheduled time, when you know you usually start to get more short of breath, as above OR on an "as needed" or "PRN" basis.

Most people do not want to take any more medication than necessary, which is completely understandable. However, many people view their rescue inhaler as a last resort to be used only "in case of emergency". Again, while we understand why someone might feel this way, we don't necessarily agree with that approach for several reasons.

First, by the time you reach that dreaded "code red" situation, you are probably already in too much distress to take the medication properly. In addition, with a little planning, you can use the principle of supply and demand to get the most benefit from your rescue medication and maximize your ability throughout the day.

For example, if you know that you will be going outside in the cold and cold causes your airways to constrict, you could take your rescue medication 15-30 minutes beforehand so that your airways are maximally dilated before you go out. The same can be done before exercise. By taking your rescue medication 15-30 minutes before beginning exercise, you can ensure that you will get the most benefit from your workout. The same can be said for showering, many people have a very difficult time in the shower. By taking your rescue medication 15-30 minutes before showering, you decrease your chances of getting into trouble. By stacking the odds in your favor, you wind up working smarter, not harder.

How NOT to Use Your Rescue Medication

We have given you some "dos" related to using your short-acting (rescue) medication. There are also a few important "don'ts".

Do not overuse your rescue medication. If you find yourself using your rescue medicine more frequently than every 4-6 hours, contact your physician because something is wrong. In fact, using these medications too frequently can actually make you "refractory" (i.e. resistant) to their effects. Taking your medications too frequently saturates the chemical binding sites in your lungs, meaning *they will not work.* This is akin to stepping on the gas too often and flooding your engine. This is especially true if you are also taking long-acting medications as well, which should significantly reduce the need to take your rescue medication, which leads to our next point.

Do not take your short-acting (rescue) medication before your long-acting medication. For example, if you are taking a long-acting beta-2 agonist PLUS a short-acting beta-2 agonist as a rescue medication. DO NOT take the SABA at the same time as or less than 2 hours before the LABA.

Many people take their short-acting bronchodilator before they take their long-acting bronchodilator (e.g. anticholinergic or beta-2 agonist), because they incorrectly believe that the short-acting bronchodilator opens up or "primes" the airways so that you get better delivery of the long-acting bronchodilator. Nothing could be farther from the truth. In fact, taking a short-acting medication before taking a long-acting medication in the same class can actually cause the exact opposite effect, requiring more frequent (but less effective) use of the rescue inhaler.

Both short-acting and long-acting beta-2 agonists bind to the same receptor sites, as short-acting and long-acting anticholinergics bind to the same receptor sites. Therefore, if you take the short-acting medication first, you will be taking up binding sites that should be reserved for the long-acting medications. As a result, this can make the long-acting medications less effective and again, actually increase the need for the short-acting ones.

Finally, if you do feel the need to take your rescue medication AFTER you have already taken your long-acting medications, try to wait AT LEAST one hour after the long-acting medication. This gives the long-acting medication time to bind to their appropriate binding sites without competition. If you cannot wait at least the minimum 4 hours before taking your rescue medication, please speak to your doctor as this indicates that your disease is poorly controlled on your current regimen.

Use the timeline below to plan out your daily medication schedule.

My Medication Schedule

6 AM ____

8 AM ____

10 AM ____

12 Noon ____

2 PM ____

4 PM ____

6 PM ____

8 PM ____

10 PM ____

12 Mid ____

"How do I use this thing?"

Patients often tell me that their "medications don't work" or that "they aren't doing anything" for them. When I ask them to show me how they take the medication, I can tell immediately why they are not seeing (or feeling) any results. The reason is that the medication is not going into their airways. Instead, it is winding up in the air, on their tongue or in their mouth and throat. This will not work.

This is like having a headache and instead of carefully placing the Tylenol in your mouth; someone throws it at you from across the room. Sure, every once in a while, one might wind up going in, but this technique would likely not do much to help your headache. This may seem like a ridiculous example, but it's actually the same with your pulmonary medications. If they don't get into your airways and lungs, they will not work.

For that reason, how you take your medication has a very significant impact on the effectiveness of the drug. If you want your medication to get into your lungs (which you do), you need to use them properly. The goal is not to haphazardly spray the medication somewhere in the direction of your mouth. It's not Binaca breath spray. Instead, the goal is for the medication to *join with* a big whoosh of air so that it can be delivered as far down into the lungs as possible.

MEDICATION DELIVERY DEVICES

Metered Dose Inhaler (MDI)

Using a Metered Dose Inhaler WITHOUT a Spacer:

- **Remove the cap from the inhaler and shake the MDI vigorously for 15 seconds.** This evenly disperses the medication throughout the entire solution that it is carried in, ensuring that the amount of medication in each 'puff' will be a consistent dose.

- **Before placing the inhaler in your mouth, take a deep breath in through your nose and out gently through pursed lips, emptying the lungs as much as you can.** This will ensure that you will be able to take the deepest breath possible in order to breathe the medication deep into your lungs.
- **Place the inhaler in between your teeth with your lips sealed firmly around the mouthpiece OR hold the inhaler 2 inches from your mouth with your mouth open.** Ideally, you should always use a spacer with gas-powered MDI's. See below for information on using a spacer.
- **As you start to breathe in, squeeze the device, discharging the medication and breathe in as slowly and deeply as you can.**
- **Hold your breath for a slow count of 5-10 seconds.** This allows the medication droplets to "fall out" of the air you brought it in with and to settle on the airway surfaces where it can make contact with the binding sites.
- **Blow out gently through pursed lips.**
- **Repeat as prescribed.**

IMPORTANT: If you are supposed to take a second puff, the entire sequence must be repeated including shaking the container. Wait approximately 1-2 minutes in between puffs to give the first puff a chance to start working and give you a chance to catch your breath.

Spacers

One of the greatest ironies about inhaled pulmonary medications is that as a group, people with respiratory disease have the most difficulty coordinating their breathing. Yet, properly and effectively inhaling medications requires a very high level of coordination of breathing! For those who use gas-powered MDI's, that's where a spacer device comes into play. A spacer is a device that is used with your MDI in order to ensure that you are actually getting the medication *and* that it is going where we want it to go: into your airways and lungs. Spacers eliminate the timing and breath-coordination difficulties by receiving the medication mist and holding it suspended in the air within the device. This allows you to more easily take in the slow deep breath we talked about above *and* get the most medication into your lungs when you *do* breathe in. Many also make a noise to let you know if you are breathing in too quickly. If you do use an MDI, I would *strongly* recommend that you use a spacer as often as possible.

Using a Metered Dose Inhaler WITH a Spacer:

- **Remove the cap from the inhaler and shake the MDI vigorously for 15 seconds.** This evenly disperses the medication throughout the entire solution that it is carried in, ensuring that the amount of medication in each 'puff' will be a consistent dose.
- **Remove the cap from the spacer and insert the MDI.**
- **Before placing the inhaler in your mouth, take a deep breath in through your nose and out gently through pursed lips, emptying the lungs as much as you can.** This will ensure that you will be able to take the deepest breath possible in order to breathe the medication deep into your lungs.
- **Place the spacer in between your teeth with your lips sealed firmly around the mouthpiece.**

- **As you start to breathe in, squeeze the device, discharging the medication and breathe in as slowly and deeply as you can.**
- **Hold your breath for a slow count of 5-10 seconds.** This allows the medication droplets to "fall out" of the air you brought them in with and to settle on the airway surfaces where it can make contact with the binding sites.
- **Blow out gently through pursed lips.**
- **Repeat as prescribed.**

IMPORTANT: If you are supposed to take a second puff, the entire sequence must be repeated including shaking the container. Wait approximately 1-2 minutes in between puffs to give the first puff a chance to start working and give you a chance to catch your breath.

Dry Powder Inhalers (DPI)

There are a number of medications on the market that use devices that are categorized as dry-powder inhalers. As the name indicates, as compared to a liquid, the inhaled medication is in the form of a dry powder. In general, they work similarly to MDI's. However, each device has a slightly different method of releasing the medication. Another difference is that when taking a DPI, you want to inhale the medication more quickly as opposed to slow and steady as you do with an MDI.

Using a Dry Powder Inhaler:

- **Open or Remove the cap from the inhaler and release the dose of medication into the device.** This will vary depending upon the device.

- **Before placing the inhaler in your mouth, take a deep breath in through your nose and out gently through pursed lips, emptying the lungs as much as you can.** This will ensure that you will be able to take the deepest breath possible in order to breathe the medication deep into your lungs.
- **Place the inhaler in between your teeth with your lips sealed firmly around the mouthpiece.**
- **Breathe in fairly quickly and as deeply as possible.**
- **Hold your breath for a slow count of 5-10 seconds.** This allows the medication to "fall out" of the air you brought them in with and to settle on the airway surfaces where it can make contact with the binding sites.
- **Blow out gently through pursed lips. Do not exhale into the device.**
- **Repeat as necessary until all medication is used.**

Respimats

NOTE: Respimats differ from one company and medication to another. *Some* must be primed. Others don't need priming. Be sure to carefully read the instructions that come with your specific Respimat.

Using a Respimat:

- **Hold the Respimat upright.**
- **Turn the base toward the arrow until you hear a click, releasing the medication.** This also loads the "spring – which is set to release and propel the medication out of the canister.
- **Open or Remove the cap from the Respimat.**

- **Take a deep breath in through your nose. Then, breathe out through pursed lips, emptying the lungs as much as you can.** This will ensure that you will be able to take the deepest breath possible in order to breathe the medication deep into your airways and lungs.
- **Place the inhaler in between your teeth with your lips sealed firmly around the mouthpiece.**
- **As you start to breathe in, press the button, discharging the medication and breathe in as slowly and deeply as you can.**
- **Hold your breath for a slow count of 5-10 seconds.** This allows the medication droplets to "fall out" of the air you brought them in with and to settle on the airway surfaces where it can make contact with the binding sites.
- **Blow out gently through pursed lips. Do not exhale into the device.**
- **Repeat as necessary.**

Handihalers, Breezhalers, Neohalers, Rotohalers, Oh, My!

There are also several other delivery devices including Handihalers, Breezhalers, Neohalers, Rotohalers and I am sure there will be others. It is crucial that you read all instructions very carefully and if there is something that you are unsure of, be sure to check with your doctor, pharmacist or other health care professional. If possible, ask them to demonstrate and watch you do it to make sure you are using it properly.

Nebulizers

People who struggle to use MDI's, DPI's, Respimats, Handihalers, Breezhalers, Neohalers, or Rotohalers may benefit from using a nebulizer, instead. A nebulizer is a device that aerosolizes the medication and delivers it over a longer period of time, allowing you to breathe in a more relaxed manner, over several minutes. The other benefit is that the medication starts to work immediately, allowing for deeper and deeper breaths and wider distribution of the medication throughout your airways as you continue the treatment. There are a variety of different nebulizer devices available including ones that are powered by a compressor and hand-held ultrasonic devices, among others.

Using a Nebulizer:

- **Wash your hands.**
- **Sit in a relaxed position.**
- **Place the mouthpiece in between your teeth with your lips sealed firmly around the mouthpiece.**
- **Turn the nebulizer on.**
- **Take slow, deep breaths in and out of your mouth until medication is finished.** Hold your breath for a count of 5 to 10 every several breaths to allow the medication to fall out of the air in your lungs.

When finished using the nebulizer, be sure to clean it according to the instructions that come with it. Failure to properly clean and maintain your nebulizer can lead to inefficient function or failure and puts you at increased risk of infection.

And there you have it, Ladies and Gentlemen; the Who, What, When, Where and Why of how to get the maximum benefit from your medications.

Now go get ‘em!

CHAPTER 7
EXERCISE

"A body at rest will remain at rest and a body in motion will remain in motion, unless acted upon by an external force."
– Sir Isaac Newton's First Law of Motion

One of my absolute core beliefs is that when it comes to health and wellness, exercise is by far, one of, if not *the* single best, most effective lifestyle change you can make and one of the most powerful tools to improve your health as well as your overall quality of life. By going from sedentary to active or from active to more active, you can *reasonably* expect to see improvements in many of your individual physical and physiological systems, as well as your body as a whole, and dare I say, your mind and spirit as well. I realize that this may seem a bit cliché (which I usually hate) or new age (which I don't hate at all), but in this case, it happens to be true.

A basic fact of *most* exercise programs for *most* people is that you will generally get out of it what you put into it. Another basic fact is that not all people are created equal. Therefore, not all programs will have the same impact on everyone.

For all of these reasons, I would be doing you a tremendous disservice if I were to tell you "this is exactly what *you* should be doing". Instead, I will teach the *principles* that have been most successful for the greatest number of patients at the Pulmonary Wellness & Rehabilitation Center. I'll also show you how to evaluate and make adaptations to your own program in order to ensure maximum safety, effectiveness and hopefully, maybe even a little fun.

PROFESSIONAL AND LEGAL DISCLAIMER: As I mention time and time again, my patients' safety is my first, second and third priority. Therefore, as with any lifestyle change, please *do not* begin *any* exercise program under the misguided pretense that "Noah told me to do this" or "Noah told me to do that." I did not, I am not and I will not tell you what *you* should do. So please, regardless of *anything* you read in this book, *always* discuss *any* lifestyle changes you plan to make with your physician before you begin.

Why Exercise?

Exercise has the ability to increase not only the pumping power of your heart and the efficiency with which your body utilizes oxygen (which pretty much, everyone knows) but also, the mechanics of your respiratory system and lung function (which, not everyone believes). Exercise also strengthens your skeletal muscles, increases your bone density, reduces body fat, regulates blood sugar and blood pressure, elevates your mood, etcetera, etcetera, etcetera. And, it makes you feel good! Maybe not at the exact moment you're doing it, but when done right, the benefits of exercise will far outweigh any minor discomfort you may experience in carrying out your actual workout.

Notice that I said *done right*, because like anything else; if you do it wrong—and there are *plenty* of people doing it wrong—not only will you not achieve the best results, but you could actually do yourself harm.

"The First Cut is the Deepest"

I often say that the first minute in the gym is the hardest—in other words, just getting there. So, go. When I used to work at NYU, I had a daily dilemma. Every afternoon, when I arrived at the corner of 34th Street and Third Avenue, I could either continue 1 more block up 34th Street and go to the gym, or I could turn right on Third Avenue and go home to watch TV, eat, and sleep. It was quite literally a daily struggle. So, trust me. *I understand.* After all, if exercising were fun and easy, everyone would be in great shape.

However, for most people, once they're actually at the gym (or physical therapy, or pulmonary rehab), they usually don't seem to mind it so much and they almost always feel better afterward. So, like Nike says, "Just do it." I would take that axiom a step further and say, "Just do something"—*anything*, almost because it *almost* doesn't matter which type of exercise you choose (within reason), as long as you do some form of activity every day. In other words, show up. So, get up out of your chair or off the couch and haul your butt over to the gym, park, mall, rehabilitation center, your basement or living room, or wherever else it is that inspires you to move your body.

A basic rule is that your body gets good at doing what you ask it to do. So, if you ask yourself to sit on the couch, eating donuts and flipping the remote (ooh, that sounds nice), that's what your body will get good at. If this is the "*workout*" you choose, you will find yourself "*rewarded*" with increased stores of adipose tissue (fat); decreased muscle size, strength and efficiency; increased shortness of breath; and a decrease in your overall aerobic capacity along with thinning bones and a whole host of *negative* adaptations to inactivity. A sedentary lifestyle is also a well-known *modifiable* risk factor for atherosclerosis and coronary artery disease (CAD).

Conversely, if you ask your body to get moving—whether you choose to walk, run, cycle, swim, participate in a formal pulmonary rehab program or any one of the many other potential exercise options—your body will get good at doing those activities, and you will soon find yourself *really* rewarded with *decreased* fat stores, *increased* muscle size, strength and efficiency; *decreased* shortness of breath; and an *increase* in your overall aerobic capacity, along with *increased* bone density and a whole host of *positive* adaptations to activity. In addition, an active lifestyle *reduces* your risk for atherosclerosis and coronary disease. I vote for what's behind door number two.

In this chapter, I will explain how to implement these practices safely and effectively, and as hip-hop legend, Biggie Smalls once said, "go from negative to positive, and it's all good." With that in mind, my goals for this chapter include:

1. To help you understand how to assess your current (baseline) fitness level.
2. To help you start an exercise program that will be the safest and most effective program *for you.*
3. To help you stay motivated and on course with your program.

Let's go!

Exercise Versus Activity

When I ask people whether or not they exercise, they often tell me that while they don't participate in any type of "formal" exercise program, they are "*very active*." When I inquire further, they usually tell me they do a lot of cleaning or grocery shopping (or some other activity of daily living).

Don't get me wrong—it's great that you're doing these things. However, most people require more than this type of basic everyday activity to achieve the maximum benefit from exercise. Therefore, for the purposes of this chapter, while we will include these daily tasks in your overall activity count, we will not consider them "exercise."

In most cases, your program should almost always include a more formal (or at least somewhat *structured*) exercise regime in which you exercise solely for the sake of exercise, regardless of your starting point. In addition, in order for your exercise program to be the most effective (or even effective at all) certain parameters must be followed.

I often ask people to think of their health as a savings account. Using this analogy, every time you do something good for yourself, it's like putting money in the bank. In this case, we are talking about exercise or activity, but this can also include things like meditating, getting a massage, eating a healthy meal, *throwing away those cigarettes*, or any number of things you can do to take better care of yourself.

Conversely, every time you do something that is not so healthy (or downright unhealthy), like spending the whole day in front of the TV, eating a box of cookies, or smoking a cigarette, think of that as making a withdrawal and in some extreme cases, *hemorrhaging* money.

In the same way that your financial goal is to accumulate as much wealth as possible, the same should be true with respect paid to your "health wealth." It is also important to realize that some deposits will be greater than others, meaning that some activities will be more valuable and produce greater benefits than others.

As an example, going for a 20-minute walk will be more valuable than washing the dishes. That being said, every little bit helps and I would never want to discourage you from participating in any activity that you want (or need) to do (like washing the dishes).

Another thing to realize is that not every day is created equal. Some days will definitely be better than others. This can be dependent upon many, many factors, like the weather, whether or not you've had a good night's sleep, what or how much you've eaten (or not eaten), and a whole host of other potential factors, some of which will vary significantly from individual to individual and some that will be more universal. This is true regardless of whether you have a pulmonary condition or not.

So, if you happen to be having a particularly bad day, maybe you will only be able to deposit a dollar or a quarter or even a penny. This is still better than nothing. Except in rare instances, doing something, no matter how small, will *always* be better than doing nothing. In fact, as one of my yoga instructors says: "as long as you're giving 100% effort, you're still getting 100% of the benefit." Thanks, Stephanie! On the flip side, on the days that you feel great, you can take advantage of it by increasing your activity. On these days, since you're feeling particularly flush, perhaps you can deposit a fiver, a ten or even a twenty-dollar bill.

Activity, Inactivity, and Shortness of Breath

As you know by now, the efficiency with which your body utilizes oxygen depends on three main systems: the respiratory system, or the ability of your lungs to move air in and out; the cardiovascular system, or the ability of your heart to pump blood; and the muscular or musculoskeletal system, the ability of your skeletal muscles to extract and utilize oxygen from the blood. The more active you are, the more efficient each of these systems will become (and vice versa). The less active you are, the less efficient each of these systems will become.

In light of these facts, patients often describe the *dyspnea cycle* as a "downward spiral" or they tell me that they are "going downhill". The good news is that in the same way that you can "spiral downhill," your body's abilities can actually improve with activity, and in many, if not most cases, you can actually start to "*spiral uphill*" again.

Please keep in mind that there are thousands of opinions out there based on people's personal and professional experiences with exercise, as well as a multitude of other factors that go into promoting one form, philosophy, or product versus another. In fact, it can be dizzying listening to the "experts" argue over which is "the best" form of exercise and how it should be done. I will provide you with what I believe is the most beneficial information based upon 25 years of experience working with cardiovascular and pulmonary patients, both at NYU's Rusk Institute of Rehabilitation Medicine and the Pulmonary Wellness & Rehabilitation Center. It's up to you to take it from there.

In order to help you gain a clear understanding of the factors involved in maximizing your exercise program, I have divided this exercise chapter into three parts. The first section will discuss general principles of exercise, like frequency, intensity, type and time of exercise (FITT). This will provide you with a general overview of which variables are important in establishing the most effective program for you and how each one can be adjusted to give you the most effective workout.

The second part will address what we call exercise testing and prescription. In this portion, I'll explain the basic principles of establishing a baseline and creating the most effective program for you.

Finally, I will walk you through the process I follow when I see a new patient and show you how we create individualized exercise programs based on the data obtained during our initial meeting.

The FITT Principle

When people discuss exercise programs, we often hear about the *FITT principle*, which stands for *Frequency* of exercise, *Intensity* of exercise, *Type* of exercise and *Time* or duration of exercise. In other words how often should I exercise, how hard should I exercise, what exercises should I do and how long should I do them for? Basically, these are the four modifiable variables that can be adjusted depending upon your current fitness level and your desired outcome. First, I will discuss each of these variables individually and then I will put them together into sample workouts for you as they specifically relate to people living with lung disease, so that you can begin to develop your own personal exercise program.

Part of the problem is that exercise recommendations are often too general in nature. Also, let's be honest. I can tell you whatever I want to tell you and regardless of what I recommend, you can still choose to do (or not do) whatever you want. For example, I can say "use the exercise bike three times per week for 45 minutes" but if you hate the exercise bike, then you're probably not going to do it. Trust me when I say that I have seen (and owned) many very expensive clothes hangers in my time. For that reason, I've instead chosen to describe several different options for you as well as to explain what you can reasonably expect from each, and then, allow you to decide what works best *for you.*

FREQUENCY OF EXERCISE

When the question of how often people should exercise comes up, you will often hear a wide range of recommendations from the once a week "miracle" to what seems like eight days a week. For general health and fitness benefits, you will most often hear people say three to five days per week (which is *approximately* what I will say).

In my experience, people feel best and make the most progress when they do *some form* of exercise every day or *almost* every day. This doesn't mean that every day has to be spent in the gym or at pulmonary rehab. In fact, it shouldn't. I often tell people that "you do rehab you so you can live your life"—not the other way around.

Here is an exercise myth buster: Many people believe that the body requires a full day of rest between workouts. This is not actually the case. In fact, daily exercise is even more important for people who are sicker or more physically deconditioned. This may seem counterintuitive. However, there are several strong arguments in favor of daily exercise:

1. Depending upon how weak or deconditioned you are; you may only be able to tolerate very short periods of low-intensity exercise. Since these initial workouts will be shorter and less intense, your body will require less recovery time in between workouts.
2. Because these workouts will be shorter and less intense you will need to do them more frequently in order to gain some momentum. Remember that a body at rest will remain at rest. Also, if you think back to your savings account, because you are making smaller deposits, you will need to make more of them if you want to see your savings grow. Therefore, you may need to do your exercise every day or in some cases, more than once per day. For example, a patient in the hospital might need to go for a walk two to three times per day or every couple of hours in order to build up their strength and endurance. Likewise, a homebound patient may need to do their chair exercises two to three times per day or walk around their living room once an hour.
3. As I mentioned previously, your body gets good at doing what you ask it to do. Therefore, you have to ask your body to become more active by exercising more frequently. This will offset the

> amount of time spent lying in bed and counteract the detrimental effects of inactivity. Think about trying to get a stalled car moving. Initially, it takes a much greater push to get it moving, and then momentum kicks in. It's similar with exercise.

At PWRC, our patients participate in formal cardiopulmonary exercise sessions two, three, or four days per week, depending upon their particular condition. As you get stronger and your workouts become longer and more intense, you may need more recovery time or to vary the types of workouts in order to prevent injury, ensure your safety and make sure you are getting the maximum benefit out of your program. As I mentioned, people do best when they do *some form* of exercise every day or *almost* every day but I am also a realist and I know that sometimes life can get in the way. However, here is what you can *reasonably* expect from various frequencies of exercise:

One Time Per Week:

The *minimum* number of times per week that we allow patients to attend our program is *two*. There are specific reasons for this. First of all, by exercising only one day per week, you cannot reasonably expect to see *any* physical or physiologic changes. In other words, from a benefit perspective, exercising one time per week is like exercising *zero* times per week. In fact, you may even do yourself harm when you do exercise because your body is not used to what essentially boils down to a random activity, increasing your risk of either musculoskeletal injury or a cardiovascular event.

Two Times Per Week:

The *majority* of our patients attend our cardiopulmonary exercise sessions two times per week for an hour to an hour and a half per session. I know this may sound like a lot of exercise, but there are rest breaks in between each exercise and as I mentioned, the program is individualized to meet each patient's needs and ability. Now, I've also said that people do best when they do some form of exercise almost every day. For that reason, I'm hesitant to explain this next point. However, *done right, it is possible* to make gains in strength and aerobic capacity by exercising two times per week.

If you plan to work out two times per week, depending upon the length of each session, my recommendation is to focus primarily on aerobic exercise with a secondary strength component built in *if time allows* and *only* if it doesn't take anything away from your aerobic exercise. As I have mentioned previously, in addition to being the most important component for people living with pulmonary disease, aerobic exercise will still give you some degree of strength, flexibility and balance benefits as well.

If you are going to workout two times per week, I would suggest Monday and Thursday, Tuesday and Friday or Wednesday and Saturday. This schedule gives you the most equal spacing and balance between exercise and rest between each workout. Since you would likely be doing the same or similar workout each day, your schedule might look something like this:

Sunday	Monday	Tuesday	Wednesday	Thursday	Friday	Saturday
	A			A		

Three Times Per Week:

By adding that third day of exercise, not only are you increasing the overall dosage by 50%, you are also increasing the potential variety of your workout by adding specific strength training exercises, either within each workout or using the third day to focus on areas other than aerobics such as strength training, flexibility, or balance exercises.

If you are going to workout three times per week, I would suggest Monday-Wednesday-Friday or Tuesday-Thursday-Saturday. Again, this gives you the most equal spacing and balance between exercise and rest in between each workout. Because you'll be including an additional day of exercise, I would recommend either doing the same workout on all three days (Option 1) OR developing two separate workouts depending upon your individual needs and goals and alternating them (Option 2). If you choose Option 2, you will be doing each workout three times in every two-week cycle.

Option 1

Sunday	Monday	Tuesday	Wednesday	Thursday	Friday	Saturday
	A		A		A	

Option 2

Sunday	Monday	Tuesday	Wednesday	Thursday	Friday	Saturday
	A		B		A	
	B		A		B	

Four Times Per Week:

By adding a fourth day of exercise, you are now potentially doubling the dose of a twice-per-week program and also further increasing the potential variety of your routine. This lends itself to a very nice split program in which you do workout A two times per week and workout B two times per week. In this type of a routine, you would benefit by splitting your workout by exercise or muscle group. For example, during workout A, you might prioritize the treadmill and during workout B, the elliptical machine or Nu-Step. This gives you the greatest variety of exercise and also, ensures that each muscle group has adequate rest, decreasing your chances of overtraining or developing an overuse injury. Since you'll be doing the same or similar workout twice per week, your schedule might look something like this:

Sunday	Monday	Tuesday	Wednesday	Thursday	Friday	Saturday
	A	B		A	B	

Five Times Per Week:

By exercising five times per week, you are giving yourself a great deal of benefit in terms of dosage and variety of exercise. That being said, keep in mind that as we start increasing the number of workouts per week, we are also diminishing the number of rest days and potentially, your body's ability to recuperate in between workouts. For that reason, I would *not* recommend doing more than five *formal* workouts per week.

Because you will be including an additional day of exercise, I would recommend doing Workout A on three alternating days and Workout B on two days in between and then reversing them the following week. If you choose this option, you'll do each workout five times in every two-week cycle.

	Sunday	Monday	Tuesday	Wednesday	Thursday	Friday	Saturday
Week 1		A	B	A	B	A	
Week 2		B	A	B	A	B	

Six or Seven Times Per Week:

If you still want to be active on the other days, I would suggest doing something that you truly enjoy like walking, swimming or taking your grandkids to the park as opposed to a formal regimented gym or rehab workout.

NOTE: It is *crucial* that you listen to your doctor, your health care team, and *your body*. Always start with the minimum effective dose of exercise—in this case, two days per week—before gradually increasing in order to greatly minimize the chance of any musculoskeletal injury, cardiovascular event, or any other adverse effect that could potentially be associated with exercise.

INTENSITY OF EXERCISE

When it comes to the intensity of exercise, we are referring to how hard you are working or the percentage of your maximum (actual or predicted) workload. There are many ways to measure the intensity of your workout including both objective and subjective criteria. *Objective* criteria include those that can be observed, counted, measured, or otherwise quantified by an instrument or outside source such as heart rate, blood pressure, or oxygen saturation. However, the objective data is only half the story.

Subjective criteria include things like your personal perception of what you are feeling and experiencing internally. The subjective data—what you're feeling with respect to breathlessness, rating of perceived exertion, as well as any other symptoms or sensations you may be experiencing—is equally, *if not more* important in gaining a complete understanding of your condition. By taking all of these factors into consideration, we are able to maximize your safety and ensure the greatest effectiveness within each workout.

Objective Measures of Exercise Intensity

Maximum Heart Rate:

One of the most common ways that we can represent the intensity of exercise or activity is by the percentage of your maximum heart rate (HR

Max%). This method is often very effective, but it can also be equally ineffective depending upon how the numbers are derived. Let me explain why I say this.

Your maximum heart rate is the maximum number of times your heart can beat per minute when you are working at your highest level of exertion or activity. It is based primarily on your age and level of conditioning. As a general rule, as we age, our maximum heart rate decreases and as another general rule, the more conditioned we are, the lower your heart rate will be, both at rest and at any given workload.

The Theoretical, The Actual and The "Actual" Actual

Your *theoretical* age-predicted maximum heart rate is most often calculated using the formula 220 minus your age (220-age). For example, a 60-year-old person has a *theoretical* age-predicted maximum heart rate of 160 beats per minute (bpm).

However, it is important to understand that this age-predicted formula for maximum heart rate is a theoretical *approximation* based upon *general* population data. It is not an individually established calculation based on your or any one person's distinct set of medical, physical, or other physiological characteristics.

Furthermore, this approximation should only be used as a predictor in "normal, healthy individuals." It does not apply to and therefore, should not be used for "high risk" populations, including anyone with any type of cardiovascular, pulmonary, metabolic, or otherwise significant medical condition that might impair normal exercise physiology or compromise safety.

In clinical or medical settings, we cannot and should not be using the theoretical maximum heart rate. Instead, we need to establish an *actual* maximum heart rate for each individual patient. For that reason, it is strongly recommended that the patient undergo a comprehensive cardiovascular workup prior to beginning an exercise or rehabilitation program, especially in these special cardiopulmonary populations.

At a *minimum*, depending on the number and degree of risk factors, some type of clinical exercise evaluation or stress test (preferably, with an echocardiogram) should be performed in order to determine the patient's *actual* maximum heart rate as well as to establish safe parameters for exercise. However, here is where things get interesting (and tricky and confusing). When it comes to pulmonary patients, even the actual maximum heart rate does not always apply either.

During a traditional stress test, the exercise would typically be terminated when the patient reaches what we call a *hemodynamic* or *physiologic endpoint*. Usually, these endpoints are based on the patient's age, gender, fitness level, and medical condition, particularly the presence of any potential cardiac risk factors. These endpoints most frequently include heart rate (HR) or pulse in beats per minute (bpm), heart rhythm via electrocardiogram (ECG or EKG), blood pressure (BP) in millimeters of mercury (mm Hg), aerobic capacity or peak oxygen consumption (VO_2 max) and in the case of pulmonary patients, oxygen saturation (O_2 Sat%).

The test is usually stopped once any one of these pre-determined endpoints is reached, or for any number of other reasons including chest pain, tachycardia (high heart rate), hyper- or hypotension (high or low blood pressure respectively), equipment malfunction, or at the patient's request.

However, it is important to understand that patients with pulmonary disease are often prevented from reaching their true maximum because they are limited by shortness of breath and/or lower extremity fatigue, long before they reach any of these physiologic endpoints. For example, that 60-year-old man might have to stop the test because he is too short of breath to continue even though his heart rate is only 120 as opposed to his age-predicted maximum heart rate of 160. In this scenario, instead of an *actual* maximum heart rate, we get what we call a *symptom-limited* maximum heart rate.

In traditional cardiac rehabilitation programs, an exercise prescription might include a target heart rate (THR) somewhere between 50% and 90% of maximum, depending on the individual's medical history, their current level of conditioning and their personal health and fitness goals. However, this is not effective in a pulmonary population or in any patient who is limited by their symptoms prior to being limited by their cardiovascular condition or hemodynamic performance. Another point to make is that many of the medications used to treat pulmonary patients can have a stimulant effect. As a result, in addition to the increased work of breathing and deconditioning, pulmonary patients can sometimes have elevated heart rates, both at rest as well as during exercise.

Metabolic Equivalents (METs)

A Measure of Exercise Tolerance or Metabolic Equivalent (MET) is a unit of measure used to describe cardiovascular workload. One MET equals 3.5 ml $O_2 \cdot kg^{-1} \cdot min^{-1}$. In English, this means that for each metabolic equivalent or MET, your body utilizes 3.5 milliliters of oxygen per kilogram of body weight per minute. To take this one step further, each person's body uses a certain amount of oxygen per minute, depending upon the activity they are doing, their body weight and composition, and their fitness level.

We can determine the exact MET level at which a person is working either by direct measurement (using what we call expired gas analysis) or by using predicted values. During a cardiopulmonary stress test, the actual milliliters of oxygen that are consumed by that patient per minute are measured. When we plug that number into a formula that adjusts for that patient's weight, we are able to determine their *actual* MET level.

We can also reasonably predict the *approximate* MET level of various activities, including different treadmill intensities, based upon data that has been collected from thousands of exercise tests and activity measurements from thousands of subjects.

For every 1.0 MET (which is consistent with being at rest), a person will use 3.5 ml of oxygen per minute for every kilogram of body weight. Therefore, if a person's body weight is 50 kilograms (approximately 110 pounds), at rest or at 1.0 MET, they use 3.5 ml of oxygen per minute multiplied by 50 kg. In other words, they use 175 ml of oxygen per minute under resting conditions, or at 1.0 MET.

If that 50 kg person exercises for 1 minute and uses 350 ml of oxygen, their body uses double the amount of oxygen as it did at rest. In other words, this person was exercising at twice the level of exertion as compared to resting conditions, or 2.0 METs.

Thankfully, we have averages for each treadmill level (intensity), so we don't have to figure it out every time. Instead, you can use the treadmill MET chart and age-predicted treadmill intensities I have provided for this purpose in chapter 6: Treadmill 101.

Subjective Measures of Exercise Intensity

Rating of Perceived Exertion (RPE) Scale

Named for its creator, Dr. Gunnar Borg, the Borg Scale or Rating of Perceived Exertion (RPE) Scale is simple to use and can be an invaluable tool for creating, monitoring and modifying an exercise program. The original scale ranges from 6-20 and represents a subjective measure of how hard the person is working. A rating of 6 is equal to rest or very, very light exertion and a rating of 20 is equivalent to maximum exertion. Each number also corresponds to a description in words ranging from very, very light all the way to very, very hard.

Rating of Perceived Exertion (RPE) Scale	
6	
7	Very Very Light
8	
9	Very Light
10	
11	Fairly Light
12	
13	Somewhat Hard
14	
15	Hard
16	
17	Very Hard
18	

19	**Very Very Hard**
20	

Multiplying each number by 10 will give us an approximate heart rate range where 60 corresponds to the person's heart rate at rest and 200 corresponds to their heart rate at maximum exertion. There is also a modified version of this scale that ranges from 0-10, but in my opinion, the 6-20 scale works better and is the one we use at PWRC.

The majority of your workout should take place in the "somewhat hard" range, increasing from *fairly light* at the beginning, working up to *somewhat hard* for the majority of the workout, and finally working *hard* at the peak, followed by a short cool-down period.

Perceived Dyspnea (Breathlessness) Scale

As compared to factors that can be observed by another person, like respiratory rate or increased work of breathing, dyspnea refers to a person's own internal perception of breathlessness. Similar to the RPE Scale, the Dyspnea (Breathlessness) Scale can be used to quantify the degree of shortness of breath a person is experiencing. This scale also ranges from 6-20, where a rating of 6 corresponds to none or very, very mild breathlessness and 20 corresponds to very, very strong breathlessness.

Perceived Dyspnea (Breathlessness) Scale	
6	
7	**Very Very Mild**
8	
9	**Very Mild**

10	
11	**Fairly Mild**
12	
13	**Somewhat Strong**
14	
15	**Strong**
16	
17	**Very Strong**
18	
19	**Very Very Strong**
20	

This information can then be correlated with more objective measures, like heart rate, blood pressure and oxygen saturation in order to determine safe and effective exercise parameters.

At PWRC, we continuously monitor our patients' heart rate and rhythm by EKG and their blood pressure and oxygen saturation are measured in five-minute intervals. We can also determine the percentage of your age- and gender-predicted maximum workload you're working at. That's what we mean by objective data.

As a point of reference, below are the *general* parameters that we use with our patients. This is assuming all things being equal, which they almost never are. As an example, if someone has known heart disease or pulmonary hypertension, we might make an adjustment to the below numbers to minimize the risk of a problem. Again, to be clear, these are *general* guidelines only. *Your* guidelines and limits should come from *your* physician.

Heart Rate: We will generally allow most of our patients to go up to a *maximum* heart rate of 200 minus their age (200-age). So, as an example, if we had an 80-year-old patient, we would allow him to go to a maximum heart rate of 120. The reason we use 200 instead of 220 is that it gives us a built-in 20 beat per minute safety zone, although most people don't reach that due to other factors like SOB or fatigue.

Blood Pressure: As far as blood pressure, if you are under eighty years of age, we will generally allow your systolic blood pressure go to a *maximum* of 200 millimeters of mercury. If you are eighty years of age or older, we will generally allow your systolic blood pressure go to a maximum of 180 millimeters of mercury. We generally try to keep diastolic pressures under 95 mm Hg.

Oxygen Saturation: As far as oxygen saturation goes, we try to keep our patients at 93% plus during exercise. In many cases, this means that we have to use supplemental oxygen but in doing so, our patients are able to get a much better workout, as compared to room air and it is these more challenging workouts that lead to the greatest short- and long-term benefits.

Rating of Perceived Exertion (RPE): Again, when it comes to RPE, we generally want our patients to warm up in the "fairly light" to "somewhat hard" range, with most of the workout being in the "somewhat hard" range and "hard" range at the peak. Exercise in the "very light" or "very very light" range is too easy and exercise in the "very hard" to very very hard" range is too intense.

Perceived Dyspnea (Breathlessness): Similarly to RPE, when it comes to breathlessness, we generally want our patients to warm up in the "fairly mild" to "somewhat strong" range with most of the workout being in the "somewhat strong" range and "strong" range at the peak.

TIME (DURATION) OF EXERCISE

How much time you spend exercising is going to be dependent upon multiple factors and can vary from person to person, and sometimes even day to day. It will depend on your medical condition, your current level of fitness, and your degree of motivation (which, as you know, can be either your best friend or your worst enemy). And then there are those million and one other factors like going to work, picking up the grandkids from school, doctor's appointments, cooking and cleaning, etcetera, etcetera, etcetera. As John Lennon of the Beatles says: "Life is what happens while we're busy making other plans."

In an ideal world, we should exercise for a *minimum* of 20 minutes per day with an ultimate goal of 45 to 90 minutes per day. I know this is a big range, but it will make more sense later, when I give you sample workouts for 20 minutes, 30 minutes, 45 minutes, 60 minutes, and even a 90-minute workout for you exercise junkies.

In my experience with patients, the most effective workouts are between 30 and 60 minutes in duration with short rest breaks interspersed throughout the workout. If you can only tolerate 10 minutes of exercise (or less) at a time, you really need to be exercising two to three times per day. The good news is that there is evidence that suggests three 10-minute workouts per day are *almost* as effective as one 30-minute workout. Keep in mind that these workout times are in addition to all of the other activities you do in your daily life.

TYPE OF EXERCISE

When we talk about the type of exercise, we are referring to the broad, general categories into which exercise can be divided. For the purposes of this book and my "typical" patient, I have included the five categories that we have found to be the most beneficial for people living with pulmonary disease. These five categories include breathing retraining, aerobic exercise, strength training, flexibility exercises, and balance training.

We will consider each of these categories from the perspective of both their *physiologic* impact on the body and their *functional* impact on the individual as a whole, during everyday activity. For example, when we talk about strength training, the physiological impact involves increasing the size of the muscles and the force with which they can contract.

When we talk about the functional impact, we are referring to the application of this force during everyday activities (e.g. getting up from a chair or lifting up your grandchild). I will try to make this connection between physiologies and function whenever possible so that you have a clear understanding of how different exercises impact your everyday life. Then, you can decide which ones are most important *for you*.

Another key point is that whether it's in the physiology lab, at pulmonary rehab or in fitness magazines at the local supermarket, people often rigidly discuss and classify the types of exercise into distinct physiological and functional categories as if they somehow exist solely as independent entities and to the exclusion of all other categories. In reality, the majority of exercises and activities that we do involve a combination of two or more types of exercise.

In other words, even when you are doing what is traditionally considered to be aerobic exercise, you will still get secondary gains in strength, flexibility, and balance as well. Similarly, when doing strength training, you can also gain some aerobic and balance benefits, and finally, when you are doing stretching or flexibility exercises, you can also gain strength and aerobic benefits.

For example, walking is usually considered to be an aerobic activity, with elements of balance, strength, flexibility and breath control required as well. However, when walking uphill or climbing stairs, a greater degree of muscle force is required making it more strength-intensive. My point in mentioning this is to say that you will get at least some benefit in multiple areas during most physical activities.

With this in mind, our goal is to create a program that incorporates each of these types of exercise that will give you the maximum benefit in the most areas with the least amount of time and effort. In other words, we want you to work smarter, not necessarily harder.

BREATHING RETRAINING

Breathing retraining includes diaphragmatic breathing, pursed-lip breathing, paced breathing, and recovery from shortness of breath. Although they are covered in Chapter 3, I wanted to mention them here in the context of exercise in order to keep things in their proper perspective (and chronologic order). These techniques provide you with greater breath control, which is why they are the first thing we teach our patients during their initial exercise session.

When you first begin learning and practicing these breathing methods, the techniques themselves are the actual exercises. However, as you become more skilled in their application, you will use them as a *tool* that will allow you to do more vigorous exercise. It is this vigorous exercise that will ultimately decrease your shortness of breath, allowing you to walk more and potentially improving your lung function in the process. If you haven't done it yet, read about them, study them, practice them and use them both during your workouts and in your everyday life.

AEROBIC EXERCISE

When people hear the words "aerobic exercise" or simply, "aerobics," their minds usually conjure up images of Jane Fonda or a room full of sweaty—I mean *glowing* women—in neon spandex jumping around, flailing their arms and legs to 80's disco music—and *a few* sweaty men. While that certainly qualifies, for the purposes of this chapter, I will define aerobic exercise as *any* activity that is cardiovascular in nature or what some people refer to simply as "cardio." In most cases, aerobic exercise involves rhythmic exercises that use large muscle groups and that can be sustained for *relatively* long periods of time. They will typically be lower in intensity than anaerobic exercise. Think tortoise, rather than hare, because if the intensity of the exercise is too great, you will be unable to sustain it long enough for it to be aerobic.

For anyone living with a cardiovascular or pulmonary disease, aerobic exercise is, by far, the single most important type of exercise. Aerobic exercise helps your body become more efficient at using oxygen and you, less short of breath. This can occur by:

1. Improving the mechanics of your respiratory system, allowing you to move air in and out more efficiently.
2. Improving the ability of your heart to pump blood to the lungs and throughout all of the organs and tissues of the body.
3. Improving the efficiency with which your peripheral (or skeletal) muscles utilize oxygen, making them more efficient at extracting oxygen from the blood, and delivering waste products to the blood for removal.

In the context of our "supply and demand" conversation, aerobic exercise increases your body's oxygen supply while reducing its demand during physical activity, at rest and even while you sleep.

Examples of aerobic exercise include walking, jogging, cycling, swimming, and dancing, among others. If you're in the gym (or pulmonary rehab), cardio machines include the treadmill, stationary bicycle, upper body ergometer (UBE) and many others. To help you make the best choices for your own workout, I will take you through the pros and cons of each type and tell you what and why we do what we do with our patients.

Walking

Walking is one of the best possible exercises you can do, for a number of reasons. Most importantly, as human beings, walking is our primary mode of locomotion. If you cannot walk, this will severely limit your ability to get around and to participate in various activities of daily living, diminishing your overall quality of life. Walking can be done almost anywhere; indoors or outdoors and requires no special equipment other than comfortable clothing and a good pair of sneakers or walking shoes (and if you've seen some of the getups people work out in, you know that's not even entirely true).

Walking is multi-systemic and involves all exercise modes, not only enhancing aerobic capacity but also improving your strength, flexibility and balance and decreasing your shortness of breath in the process. It is also easily modifiable with respect to speed and duration, based on the individual.

Be sure to walk in a safe place like a gym, track, mall or supermarket. Walk where the air is clean and avoid temperature extremes. If you are in a hot climate, walk early in the morning before the sun is at its strongest, or in the evening when the sun is starting to go down. If you live in a cold environment, walk indoors if the temperature is below approximately 36 degrees. Finally, if you are supposed to be using an assistive device like a walker or cane, please do. The same goes for any prescribed orthotics, where applicable.

Jogging/Running

Jogging and running have many of the same benefits of walking, but with a few caveats. The biggest difference between walking and jogging or running is that when you walk (even quickly), you always have at least one foot on the ground. When you jog or run there is at least a brief period during each stride (actually two) when both feet (and the rest of your body) are off the ground. As a result, there is a greater mechanical load every time your foot hits the floor. These factors increase the impact and potential stress on your body, particularly the musculoskeletal system (joints, tendons, ligaments), significantly increasing your chances of injury.

Both of these activities can range from fairly mild to very vigorous, so they can potentially generate even greater benefits with respect to aerobic capacity. However, this increased intensity also comes with some increased risk, which is why we usually recommend walking instead of jogging or running for the majority of our patients.

Treadmill

The treadmill is my single favorite piece of exercise equipment for many reasons. First, the treadmill is highly effective, mainly because its intensity can be easily adjusted with respect to speed and incline, making it a consistently measurable and "dose-controllable" activity.

Second, the treadmill provides mechanical assistance to ambulation (walking) by bringing your leg backward with each stride. This reduces the amount of force needed to overcome the resistance exerted on your body by the ground. For this reason, many people can do more on the treadmill than they can when walking, which ultimately helps you do more *off* the treadmill. As a point of reference, walking on a flat surface is equivalent to walking at approximately a 2% incline on a treadmill.

Finally, and this is so important, holding on to the arm rails closes the chain, allowing the muscles of the thorax and the entire upper body (pecs, lats, traps, serratus) to work in their reverse actions, assisting the diaphragm and allowing you to breathe easier.

I will address the treadmill in much greater detail as well as give you several sample workouts in *Chapter 8: Treadmill 101*. That's how valuable I think it is.

Bicycling

Riding a bicycle is another great exercise that most people can participate in (in one form or another). As they say, "it *is* like riding a bike." The bike is a relatively versatile and user-friendly piece of equipment. Its various parameters (body position, speed and resistance) can all be modified based upon your cardio-respiratory fitness and any musculoskeletal limitations you may have, making it an effective workout tool for almost anybody.

Depending upon your body type and/or any physical or physiologic limitations you may have, you may find one bicycle to be more comfortable than another. As an example, because your back is supported, many people find the *recumbent bike* to be more comfortable and easier to use than an *upright bike*. However, this also makes the recumbent bike less physically (and metabolically) demanding than the upright bike.

Compared to the recumbent bike, there is also a strong postural component to the upright bike. In addition to the work of the lower body, the muscles of the thorax (chest, back and abdominals) have to work harder to keep you upright, balancing anterior (front) and posterior (back) and left and right to prevent you from falling over. As a result the upright bike is more physically (and metabolically) demanding than the recumbent bike.

In other words, the upright bike requires more muscle activity, thereby increasing its value as an aerobic exercise.

Another consideration in choosing one bike versus another is the impact of body position on respiratory mechanics. When you're on the recumbent bike as compared to the upright, your knees come up a bit higher, bringing your thighs closer towards your upper body, compressing the abdominal and thoracic contents. As a result, the diaphragm has less room to contract (downward) and in fact, can be pushed upwards, further increasing the intra-abdominal and intra-thoracic pressures. These increased intra-abdominal and intra-thoracic pressures further compress the lungs, making it more difficult for you to take a deep breath. This is particularly true for overweight individuals, especially if they have a lot of soft tissue (fat) in the midsection.

Using a stationary bike indoors can eliminate the risks of outdoor cycling while still allowing you to develop both strength and aerobic capacity and if we set up a fan in front of you, you can still get that nice *wind-blowing-through-your-hair* feeling as you ride.

Elliptical Machine

Another one of my favorites, the elliptical machine is one of the most popular exercise machines on the market and for good reason. The elliptical offers a very effective full-body workout with many of the same aerobic benefits as jogging or walking with far less impact on the joints. Elliptical machines can be done using only the lower body (while holding on with the arms) or upper and lower body at the same time.

It is significantly more strenuous to do both arms and legs as opposed to just using your legs and requires a greater balance and coordination. Beginners should start using the lower body only for a less intense workout.

As you feel more comfortable, you can add the arms, increasing the time and intensity as your fitness level improves. Be careful especially when getting on and off the machine.

Nu-Step

The Nu-Step is a semi-recumbent/recumbent cross trainer that combines forward and back arm motion (like the elliptical), with an up and down stepping motion in the legs (like a stepper), all in a seated or semi-reclining position. One of the greatest benefits of this type of design is that people of all fitness levels can use it, even if they are not capable of full weight bearing. The Nu-Step is extremely comfortable and consistently a favorite among patients.

Upper Body Ergometer (UBE)

The upper body ergometer (UBE) or "arm bike" is essentially a bicycle that you pedal with your arms. In most cases, you can pedal forwards or backward and the resistance can be adjusted in order to increase or decrease the tension, increasing or decreasing the intensity of the workout. The UBE is one of the best exercise machines on the market and almost always the first exercise we introduce our patients to in their initial session.

As human beings, we conduct the majority of activities in front of us. As a result, the muscles on the front of the body are typically stronger (and consequently tighter) than those on the back, which are usually weaker (and looser). This muscle imbalance can lead to that round-shouldered, forward-bending posture that is so common as we age and even more so in people with respiratory disease.

For this reason, we usually have people pedal backward first, while they have the most energy in order to prioritize the back muscles. In this way, we strive to restore the body's natural muscle balance and upright posture. For patients with a significant forward bend (*kyphosis*), we may have them do the entire exercise backward. The UBE is also very effective in relaxing the muscles of the upper body and the airways, increasing ribcage mobility, decreasing muscle tension and allowing you to take a deeper breath.

Arm-R-Size

Arm-R-Size is a series of 10-20 upper body movements that I believe I first learned at the UCSD pulmonary rehab program more than 20 years ago. We've been using it ever since and even added a few moves of our own. Essentially, these exercises simulate everyday activities, and each one can be done for 15-60 seconds (or more) in succession for a total exercise time of 5-15 minutes. One of the best things about this program is that it can be performed almost anywhere and doesn't require any special machines or equipment, making Arm-R-Size an invaluable addition to your overall workout or on its own.

For many people with pulmonary disease, upper body and particularly overhead (open chain) activities, are especially difficult—think washing your hair. These activities put the diaphragm and the rest of your respiratory muscles at a significant mechanical disadvantage for breathing, thereby causing you to become more short of breath and your muscles (and you) to fatigue more quickly.

Arm-R-Size can help to prevent and reverse these effects increasing the strength and endurance of your upper body, improving the mechanics of your respiratory system and desensitizing you to dyspnea, making your upper body muscles more efficient and you, less short of breath.

Swimming

Swimming is an excellent full-body, aerobic exercise for those that are able to do it. It has many of the same benefits of other aerobic exercise but creates less impact on the body due to the buoyancy of the water. However, swimming also requires a great deal of breath control and coordination and the workout will vary depending upon which stroke you choose. Be aware that people whose respiratory triggers include strong odors or irritants may have increased sensitivity to the chemicals used in pools.

Water Aerobics

Water Aerobics combine various upper and lower body movements into a full-body aerobic workout. Working out in the water uses buoyancy to assist or resist the motion, reducing impact and increasing or decreasing the resistance depending on the muscles used. Again, be aware that people whose respiratory triggers include strong odors or irritants may have increased sensitivity to the chemicals used in pools.

Aerobic Dance

Aerobic Dance is an excellent full-body workout that combines various dance movements into a full-body aerobic workout. Besides the overall health benefits for your cardiovascular fitness and endurance; aerobic dance develops balance, coordination, and flexibility. It also adds a mental component to your workout as you learn and remember new dance steps and sequences throughout the class—and *it's fun*!!!

Aerobic dance classes vary from instructor to instructor and from class to class, depending on the style and many other factors. So please be sure to choose a class that is appropriate for your fitness level.

Stairmaster/Stair Climber/Stepper

Although there are slight variations from machine to machine, the stepper allows you to utilize the same muscles as during stair climbing, which is one of the most challenging activities for people, especially if you have difficulty breathing. When you use the stepper with your hands free, you get the added benefit of working on balance and stability. However holding on increases your safety and assists with respiration by allowing the upper extremities to work in a closed chain, improving respiratory mechanics. Be careful especially when getting on and off the machine.

If you can, try to use your arms for balance and stability only. Putting too much weight on your arms significantly decreases the effectiveness of the workout and increases your chance of developing a repetitive use injury, particularly at the shoulders, elbows and wrists.

Ski Machine/NordicTrack

A ski machine is an exercise machine that, as the name suggests, is designed to replicate the act of cross-country skiing, one of the best-known aerobic workouts. Your arms and legs move through the forward and backward motion of cross-country skiing, offering a very effective full-body workout, providing many of the same benefits as jogging or walking, but with less impact on the joints.

It is significantly more strenuous to do both the arms and legs as opposed to using your legs only. It also requires greater balance and coordination. Beginners should start using the lower body only for a less intense workout. As you feel more comfortable, you can add the arms, increasing the time and intensity as your fitness level improves. Be careful especially when getting on and off the machine.

Versa-Climber

The Versa-Climber is another full-body; sitting or standing cross-trainer that combines a climbing motion of the upper body with a stepping motion of the legs. It can be used either as an upper and lower body exercise, in either seated or standing; or as a lower body exercise only, while seated. Because of the comfort of the seat and the simple stepping motion, people of all fitness levels can use it.

Rowing Machine

A Rowing Machine replicates the act of rowing a boat (or more accurately, a racing shell). Stroke! Stroke! It's used in a seated position and is a full body exercise that combines a pushing (extension) motion with the legs and a pulling (flexion) motion with the arms. The rowing machine is an excellent workout for pulmonary patients and can be very beneficial in terms of posture. However, it may be difficult for people with limited joint motion, particularly in the lower back, hips, knees and ankles.

STRENGTH TRAINING

The goal of strength or resistance training is to increase the size (mass) of your muscles and the amount of force that they can generate. This is accomplished by exercising the muscles in a way that incrementally demands greater exertion, gradually increasing the resistance over time. This can be done using a variety of exercises, including free weights (barbells, dumbbells, wrist and ankle weights), machines, therapeutic bands, isometric exercises and activities that use your own body weight as resistance.

For pulmonary patients, we usually begin with aerobic exercise and gradually add strength training once you've improved your level of aerobic conditioning sufficiently. Generally, when you can do 15 minutes of arm exercises, 15 minutes of biking or Nu-Step and 25 minutes on the treadmill, we will then begin adding specific strength training exercises. However, as mentioned earlier, even an aerobic workout will help to improve your strength. For instance, if you are very weak, and you have been inactive, then going out for a walk—which is primarily an aerobic activity—will also increase your strength.

Strengthening exercises can be divided into compound and isolation movements. Compound movements are exercises that work several different muscle groups at the same time in order to achieve a specific motion or action, whereas isolation exercises focus on one muscle or muscle group at a time. As an example, the bench press is a compound movement whose primary muscle group is the chest or pectoral muscles, but they are assisted by the muscles on the front of the shoulder (anterior deltoid) and the triceps muscles on the back of the arms. The "pectoral fly" on the other hand, focuses on the chest muscles or pectorals alone, in isolation. Ideally, you would use a combination of compound and isolation movements depending upon your personal fitness goals.

FLEXIBILITY EXERCISE

Flexibility or stretching exercises can increase your range of motion, decrease joint and muscle stiffness, and help prevent injury. While you may not need to be able to put your foot behind your head or twist yourself into a pretzel, flexibility is crucial to being able to breathe well and is essential to maintaining and improving your ability to perform a broad range of activities of daily living (ADL).

Due to poor respiratory mechanics and increased work of breathing, many people with pulmonary disease often develop muscle imbalances, particularly between the diaphragm and accessory muscles of breathing, as well as between anterior and posterior muscles of the body. Some muscles become tighter and shorter due to overuse, while others become weaker and overstretched. When this happens people may experience pain, particularly in the muscles of the neck, shoulders, back, chest and abdominals. This can further lead to skeletal adaptations of the spine and thorax.

Flexibility exercises can help correct or even prevent these imbalances, preserving diaphragmatic excursion and thoracic mobility and maximizing expansion of the lungs. In other words, flexibility exercises can help keep the respiratory muscles pliable, allowing the diaphragm to move freely and the chest and lungs to expand fully, decreasing the work of breathing.

Flexibility can also play an important role in everyday activities. For people living with a pulmonary condition, upper body, particularly overhead activities can be especially challenging. If you think back to our discussion of open chain vs. closed chain activities, you will recall that overhead (open chain) activities put the diaphragm at a significant mechanical disadvantage. In fact, people are often advised to avoid these activities altogether in the name of "energy conservation."

As an example, people are often told to avoid storing things on high shelves. However, if you don't use it, you lose it and avoiding these activities can lead to significantly decreased range of motion in the upper body, particularly, the shoulders. So, in spite of conventional wisdom, don't be so quick to avoid the activities that cause you discomfort.

Like aerobic exercise and strength training, there are several different types of flexibility or stretching exercises including static (stationary, including both active and passive), dynamic (moving), ballistic and isometric. Stretches can be used as part of your warm-up, mid-workout, or cooldown. For our purposes some combination of static and dynamic stretching would likely provide the greatest benefit while minimizing your risk of injury.

For those adventurous types who want to take your flexibility training to the next level you might consider alternative modalities such as Yoga, Pilates, Tai Chi or Qigong.

BALANCE & STABILITY TRAINING

Balance and stability training should be an essential part of any exercise program. Good balance requires the interaction of the musculoskeletal system (strength and flexibility) and the neurologic system (coordination, proprioception and sensation), among others. As we age, our balance and stability decrease, particularly if we have other conditions that diminish our strength, flexibility and neurologic function.

Improving your balance enables you to maximize the benefits of your exercise routine and overall health and wellness program. More importantly, having good balance is essential for everyday activities.

Think about the role that balance plays in the following:

- Walking on uneven surfaces
- Walking up or down stairs
- Getting in and out of bed
- Getting into and out of the shower/bath
- Bending over to pick up something from the floor
- Overhead activities such as getting something down from a high shelf or changing a light-bulb
- Getting in and out of a car
- Getting up and down from the floor

- Being able to stand while riding the bus
- Line dancing or doing the conga at your niece's wedding!

There are a broad variety of balance and stability exercises and some types may be more suitable for you than others. Balance activities can be divided into static (stationary) and dynamic (moving) activities. Some balance exercises can be performed at home, using only your own body, whereas others utilize specialized equipment such as stability balls, balance pads, foam rollers or wobble boards. In addition, there are a wealth of books, videos and classes that offer specific examples of individual or group balance exercises including alternative modalities such as Yoga, Pilates, Tai Chi or Qigong.

FINAL NOTE:

As with any exercise program, please remember that safety is our number one priority. With that in mind, please check with your physician or health care provider before beginning any exercise program.

CHAPTER 8

TREADMILL 101

"If you can't fly, then run; if you can't run, then walk, if you can't walk, then crawl, but whatever you do you have to keep moving forward."
– Martin Luther King, Jr.

When it comes to the single best exercise for cardiopulmonary patients, the treadmill is in a class by itself. There are several important reasons for this. First and foremost, as human beings, we need to walk. Second, the treadmill is highly controllable and customizable, meaning that you can set very specific workout parameters for speed, incline, and consequently, workload or MET level. Finally, the treadmill physically assists your walking and provides mechanical support for your breathing, thereby allowing you to maximize your overall workout.

Patients often remark that walking on a treadmill is different and in some ways, easier than walking outside or even from one room to the next. Notice that with each step forward, the treadmill moves your feet to the back of the belt, decreasing the resistance of the ground. As a point of reference, walking outside on a flat surface is the equivalent of walking at approximately a 2% incline on the treadmill.

Another factor is that when you fix your upper extremities by holding on to the handrails, the treadmill becomes a closed chain activity and divides the workload among four limbs instead of two. In addition, closing the chain greatly improves respiratory mechanics, allowing the muscles of your thorax; chest, back, shoulders to work in their reverse action, further assisting with ribcage elevation and overall thoracic expansion, allowing you to take a deeper breath.

Although we have touched on exercise multiple times throughout this book, I have not yet given you the specifics of treadmill exercise that you want and need. At this point, I would like to introduce some tools that will help you develop the absolute best treadmill protocol *for you* so that you can achieve the very best results within each and every workout.

As always, please do not begin any exercise program without clearing it with your doctor first, ideally after a comprehensive cardiac workup but at a minimum, some form of clinical exercise evaluation.

How Hard Should I Work Out?

When it comes to treadmill activity, patients often ask me some version of the following questions: (1) how hard should I work out, (2) what's more important: speed or incline, and (3) what's more important: time or distance. The answer is that they are all important and in fact, all directly related to and affected by one another. The longer you walk on the treadmill, the more mileage you will cover at a single speed. The faster you walk, the more mileage you will cover in the same amount of time.

However, when it comes to creating the most effective workout, that will not only produce the best results, but also have the greatest carryover to everyday life, MET Level (Measure of Exercise Tolerance or metabolic equivalent) is the most crucial (yet, frequently overlooked) factor. Also, when it comes to treadmill protocols and parameters, the MET is the great equalizer, allowing us to compare apples to apples and oranges to oranges.

As a quick review, one MET is equal to 3.5 mL of oxygen per kilogram of body weight per minute or the equivalent of your metabolic state at rest. This means that when you are at one met (think sitting quietly in a chair), your body consumes 3.5 milliliters of oxygen per minute for every kilogram (2.2 pounds) of your body weight. Activities at the two MET level would double your oxygen requirements to 7 mL of oxygen per kilogram of body weight per minute. Three METs would triple the workload and so on. You get the idea. As a point of reference, a workload of 1.1 METs to 2.9 METs is considered light, 3.0-5.9 METs is considered moderate and 6.0 METs or greater is considered vigorous activity.

Sadly, it is not only patients that are sometimes confused by this subject. Many healthcare professionals also struggle to understand how to create the most effective treadmill protocols and exercise goals for people with pulmonary conditions. In fact, if you read much of the classic literature pertaining to pulmonary rehabilitation, most people agree that patients feel less short of breath, can tolerate more activity and have a greater sense of confidence and wellbeing. However, most claims fall short of promising improved pulmonary function.

In contrast, my colleagues and I *know* that you *can* improve pulmonary function *under the right conditions*. However, as opposed to the traditional low-intensity long-duration exercise used in more traditional programs, we have consistently found that it takes moderate and high-intensity exercise if you want to improve pulmonary function. For all of these reasons, it is important for you to understand how to use MET level to your greatest advantage.

In this chapter, I will introduce you to two charts that we use at the Pulmonary Wellness & Rehabilitation Center: the Treadmill MET Chart and the American College of Sports Medicine's (ACSM) Age-Predicted Exercise Capacity (APEC Chart). Please do not be intimidated if they look complex at first. I promise after some explanation, they will make a lot of sense.

Treadmill MET Chart

The Treadmill MET Chart will tell you the MET Level for various combinations of speed and incline. The numbers across the bottom row of the chart represent speed in miles per hour (mph). The numbers in the first column on the left represent the percent incline (incline %). To determine the metabolic equivalent or MET Level, first find your speed along the bottom and then match it up with the corresponding incline. MET level is found at the intersection of speed and incline.

TREADMILL MET CHART

GRADE (% INCLINE)

15	3.8	4.1	4.4	4.7	5.0	5.3	5.5	5.8	6.1	6.4	6.7	7.0	7.2	7.5	7.8	8.1	8.4	8.7	8.9	9.2	9.5	9.8	10.1	10.4	10.6	10.9	11.2	11.5	11.8	12.1
14	3.7	4.0	4.2	4.6	4.8	5.1	5.3	5.6	5.9	6.2	6.4	6.7	6.9	7.2	7.5	7.8	8.0	8.3	8.6	8.9	9.1	9.4	9.6	9.9	10.2	10.5	10.7	11.0	11.2	11.5
13	3.6	3.9	4.1	4.4	4.6	4.9	5.1	5.4	5.6	5.9	6.1	6.4	6.6	6.9	7.1	7.4	7.7	8.0	8.2	8.5	8.7	9.0	9.2	9.5	9.7	10.0	10.2	10.5	10.7	11.0
12	3.4	3.7	3.9	4.2	4.4	4.7	4.9	5.2	5.4	5.6	5.8	6.2	6.3	6.6	6.8	7.1	7.3	7.6	7.8	8.1	8.3	8.6	8.8	9.0	9.2	9.5	9.7	10.0	10.2	10.5
11	3.3	3.5	3.7	4.0	4.2	4.5	4.7	4.9	5.1	5.4	5.6	5.8	6.0	6.3	6.5	6.7	6.9	7.2	7.4	7.7	7.9	8.1	8.3	8.6	8.8	9.0	9.2	9.5	9.7	9.9
10	3.1	3.3	3.6	3.8	4.0	4.2	4.4	4.7	4.9	5.1	5.3	5.5	5.7	6.0	6.2	6.4	6.6	6.8	7.0	7.2	7.4	7.7	7.9	8.2	8.3	8.5	8.7	9.0	9.2	9.4
9	3.0	3.2	3.4	3.6	3.8	4.0	4.2	4.4	4.6	4.8	5.0	5.2	5.4	5.6	5.8	6.0	6.2	6.4	6.6	6.8	7.0	7.2	7.4	7.6	7.8	8.0	8.2	8.4	8.6	8.8
8	2.9	3.1	3.2	3.4	3.6	3.8	4.0	4.2	4.4	4.6	4.7	4.9	5.1	5.3	5.5	5.7	5.9	6.1	6.2	6.4	6.6	6.8	7.0	7.2	7.4	7.6	7.8	7.9	8.1	8.3
7	2.7	2.9	3.1	3.3	3.4	3.6	3.8	4.0	4.1	4.3	4.5	4.7	4.8	5.0	5.2	5.4	5.5	5.7	5.8	6.0	6.2	6.4	6.5	6.7	6.9	7.1	7.2	7.4	7.6	7.8
6	2.6	2.8	2.9	3.1	3.2	3.4	3.6	3.8	3.9	4.1	4.2	4.4	4.5	4.7	4.8	5.0	5.1	5.3	5.5	5.7	5.8	6.0	6.1	6.3	6.4	6.6	6.7	6.9	7.1	7.3
5	2.5	2.6	2.7	2.9	3.1	3.2	3.3	3.5	3.6	3.8	3.9	4.1	4.2	4.4	4.5	4.7	4.8	5.0	5.1	5.3	5.4	5.6	5.7	5.9	6	6.2	6.4		6.5	6.7
4	2.3	2.5	2.6	2.8	2.8	3.0	3.1	3.3	3.4	3.5	3.6	3.8	3.9	4.1	4.2	4.3	4.4	4.6	4.7	4.9	5.0	5.1	5.2	5.4	5.5	5.7	5.8	5.9	6.0	6.2
3	2.2	2.3	2.4	2.6	2.7	2.8	2.9	3.0	3.1	3.3	3.4	3.5	3.6	3.7	3.8	4.0	4.1	4.2	4.3	4.4	4.5	4.7	4.8	4.9	5	5.2	5.3	5.4	5.5	5.6
2	2.0	2.1	2.2	2.4	2.5	2.6	2.7	2.8	2.9	3.0	3.1	3.2	3.3	3.4	3.5	3.6	3.7	3.8	3.9	4.0	4.1	4.2	4.3	4.4	4.5	4.7	4.8	4.9	5.0	5.1
1	1.9	2.0	2.1	2.2	2.3	2.4	2.5		2.6	2.7	2.8	2.9	3.0	3.1	3.2	3.3	3.4		3.5	3.6	3.7	3.8	3.9	4.0	4.1	4.2	4.3		4.4	4.5
0	1.8		1.9		2.1		2.2	2.3	2.4		2.5	2.5	2.7		2.8	2.9	3.0		3.1	3.2	3.3	3.4	3.5		3.6	3.7	3.8		3.9	4.0
	1.0		**1.2**		**1.4**		**1.6**		**1.8**		**2.0**		**2.2**		**2.4**		**2.6**		**2.8**		**3.0**		**3.2**		**3.4**		**3.6**		**3.8**	

SPEED IN MILES PER HOUR (MPH)

As an example, walking at 1.0 mph with no incline (0%) is equal to 1.8 METs. If we raise the speed to 1.6 mph, the MET level increases to 1.9 METs. If we then increase the incline to 3%, our MET level increases to 2.9 METs. You get the idea.

Here is another application. If you were to walk at 3.0 mph with a 0% incline, your level would be 3.3 METs. Now, three miles per hour may be too fast for many people (and too slow for others). However, if you were to lower that speed to 1.6 mph (approximately half), you could still reach that same 3.3 MET level by adding a 5% incline. Essentially, what this chart demonstrates is that there are many ways to accomplish the same MET level. This is an extremely valuable resource that will allow you to tailor your treadmill activity for maximum results, while individualizing the program to address and adapt to your own particular circumstances and abilities.

As an example, individuals with Spinal Stenosis, Osteoarthritis and other musculoskeletal conditions may have a harder time walking on a steep incline. In that case, you can increase the speed to achieve your target-MET level. Alternatively, if you are 4' 11" with short legs or have a neurological condition that affects your gait, maintaining a higher speed may be a challenge. In this case, you can walk at a slower speed with a higher incline to achieve your workout goal. Get it?

Age-Predicted Exercise Capacity (APEC) Chart

The ACSM's Age-Predicted Exercise Capacity (APEC) chart will tell you the percentage of exercise capacity predicted for a healthy person of your age and gender. To use this chart, first find your age on the left side. Then, take a ruler or sheet of paper and place it on your age. Then move the other side of the ruler to the MET level that you are working at (based on the treadmill MET chart). The point at which the ruler or paper intersects either the red line (for women) or the blue line (for men) represents the percentage of your age-predicted exercise capacity.

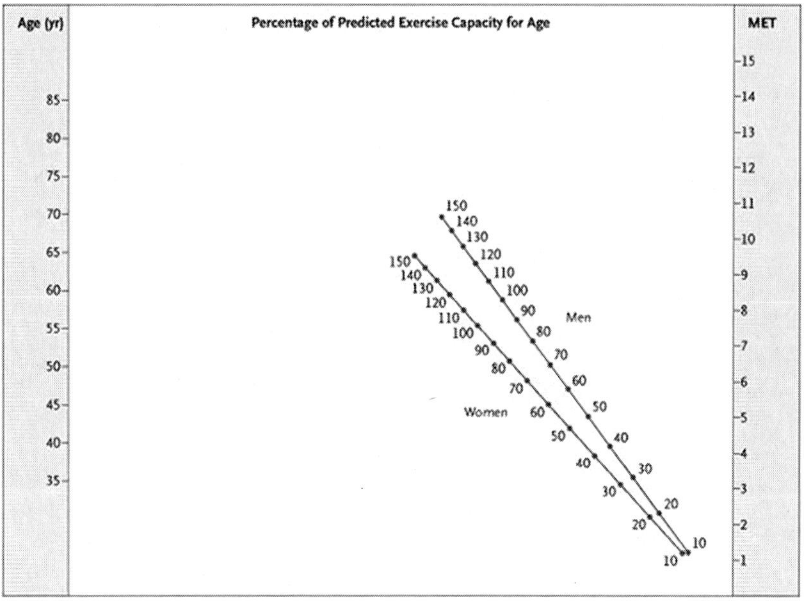

AMERICAN COLLEGE OF SPORTS MEDICINE (ACSM)
GUIDELINES FOR EXERCISE TESTING AND PRESCRIPTION

Here is another application. If you want to work out at a specific percentage of your age-predicted maximum, match up your age with the percentage of maximum that you would like to achieve and then extend the line to find out the appropriate MET level.

I encourage you to share these charts with your doctors and pulmonary rehab providers. They may or may not be aware of or practice this protocol but at The Pulmonary Wellness & Rehabilitation Center, we know that the MET counts for everything!

Creating a Treadmill Protocol

My goal with this chapter is to help you understand how to create the most effective and practical treadmill protocol *for you.* However, while I can offer you general principles and strategies, I do not know your medical history and I have not had a chance to examine you or conduct any of my own testing to assess your abilities with respect to abilities and goals. This is why it is so crucial for you to clear any exercise suggestions you may see here with your physician.

In addition, if you have any cardiovascular risk factors or are prone to desaturation (among other conditions), you should not exercise unsupervised, at least in the beginning. That being said, I am also a realist and as much as I would love to recommend a personalized exercise program for you, I realize that many readers may be setting out on this journey alone, whether it be due to lack of access to a rehab facility, insurance or other factors. Again, this is why it is crucial for you to speak with your doctor to ensure that you will be safe.

What if I don't have a Treadmill?

To be clear, I'm not saying that you can't get a good workout on a stationary bike or elliptical machine or even walking. These are all excellent alternatives. In fact, the best option is a cross training program in which you perform several different exercises within the same workout. But once again, if you want to choose the single best exercise that has the greatest chance of success, the treadmill would be my first choice, hands down.

Of course, if you do not have access to a treadmill, all is not lost. If that is your situation, then walk outside whenever possible. The MET chart can still guide you in estimating your goals. Try speeding up or slowing down and find someplace with a varied terrain where you can increase the intensity of your workout using hills and slopes for inclines.

Other Considerations

1. **Clear any and all exercise with your doctor.** I cannot emphasize this enough. Ideally, I would like every patient to have a

full physical examination as well as specific tests to assess cardiovascular risk such as a stress test with echocardiogram *at a minimum*. Under the right circumstances, exercise can be the best thing for you. Under the wrong circumstances, it can be the worst and as I have said before, when it comes to patient safety, I don't like surprises.

2. **If in doubt, refer to number 1.**

3. **Start slowly and progress gradually as tolerated.** Like Goldilocks, we like our workouts just right. However, it will always be better to err on the side of caution and underdo it rather than overdo it. Doing too much can increase your chances of an acute cardiac event or the development of an overuse injury and sometimes, you may not feel the full impact of the workout until several hours or days later. As I say to my patients: "everything will be done to your tolerance. Each time you come back and tell us that you felt well after the last session we will gradually increase your time and intensity."

4. **Think long-term and don't overdo it.** Let me put things in perspective for you. If you were to start off today walking on the treadmill at 1.0 mph and added .1 mile per hour per week, in a year, you would be walking at 6.2 mph. If you were to start off today walking on the treadmill at 0% incline and added .5% per week, in a year, you would be walking at 26% incline. Now, I am not suggesting that you will be walking at 6.2 mph with a 26% incline. I'm just trying to say you don't have to do it all in the first week.

5. **Pay attention to warning signals.** As I say to my patients: "If at any time during the workout, you feel tired, dizzy, short of breath, chest pain or pressure, or you simply want to stop the workout, let me know right away." Since, I will not be with you, don't let me know. If you are unsure, stop. This is not an excuse

not to exercise. I'm just saying that if you see any red flags, take them seriously.

6. **Push yourself whenever possible.** This may seem to contradict what I have just said in number 6. It doesn't. What I am saying is that if your life requires 5 METs, you can work out at 2 until the cows come home but your life will not be much different. Use the charts to figure out what speed, incline, and MET level you should be working at.
7. **Wear comfortable clothing and supportive sneakers or walking shoes.**
8. **Perform a gradual warm-up and cool-down.** The body doesn't like surprises. In other words, if you go from sitting in a chair to walking or running on the treadmill at your maximum capacity, your body can't tell the difference between that and getting chased by a bear and it could respond as such in the form of higher heart rates, and blood pressures, increased shortness of breath and decreased oxygen saturation. Another way to think of your workout is like a flight. You want a nice gradual takeoff, a comfortable cruising altitude and a nice smooth landing.
9. **Don't stand still when the treadmill stops.** Most people's inclination is to stand on the treadmill for a few seconds when the belt stops. However, this can cause you to become lightheaded or dizzy and in extreme cases, you could pass out. The reason for this is that when you are exercising, the heart is pumping blood to the body and the calf muscles return the blood from the lower part of the body to the heart. When you stand still, the heart is still pumping and blood can pool in your lower extremities.
10. **Rely on your instruments.** Buy a pulse oximeter and blood pressure cuff so that you can measure your vital signs (heart rate, blood pressure and oxygen saturation) before, during,

and after exercise. You cannot always go by how you feel. And again, when it comes to safety, we don't want to *assume*. We want to *know*.

11. **Do "the breathing."** Use controlled breathing techniques like abdominal breathing, pursed lip breathing and paced breathing. Time your breathing with your stepping. Breathe in, in, and blow- two, three, four (or whatever pattern works best for you).

12. **Use supplemental oxygen when necessary.** During exercise, we like our patients to be at a *minimum* oxygen saturation of 93% and we will use as much oxygen as necessary to keep them there. If you drop below 90%, you need oxygen. And given the choice, I would much rather give you more oxygen and allow you to do a bigger workout than not give it to you and have your workout be limited due to desaturation. Remember that it is these big workouts that will allow for the greatest improvements.

13. **Take your short-acting bronchodilator ("rescue inhaler") 10-15 minutes before exercise.** Of course, you need to check with your physician on this one but again, our goal is the biggest workout possible, by any means necessary. So, if this will allow you to relax the airways, open up the lungs and have a better workout, go for it!

14. **Exercise Testing and Prescription:** To be clear, all of our patients come to us by physician referral. In addition, before we begin any exercise, we do our own treadmill testing using the Bensen Treadmill Protocol, developed by one of my former colleagues, Brooke Bensen. This allows us to determine exactly where a patient is at that moment and to set up a program that is going to be safe and the most effective.

15. **Sample Workouts:** Below are several sample workouts based upon the protocols used at the Pulmonary Wellness & Rehabilitation Center. These are generic examples. They are not

specific recommendations for you or your particular situation. However, please feel free to share them with your healthcare team to help determine the appropriate starting point *for you*.

Low Intensity Protocols (1.1-2.9 METs)

Time (minutes)	**Speed** (mph)	**Incline** (%)	**MET Level**
0 (Start)	0.5	0	1.4
2	Stop		

Time (minutes)	**Speed** (mph)	**Incline** (%)	**MET Level**
0 (Start)	0.6	0	1.5
2	Stop		

Time (minutes)	**Speed** (mph)	**Incline** (%)	**MET Level**
0 (Start)	0.7	0	1.55
2	Stop		

Time (minutes)	**Speed** (mph)	**Incline** (%)	**MET Level**
0 (Start)	0.8	0	1.6
3	Stop		

Time (minutes)	**Speed** (mph)	**Incline** (%)	**MET Level**
0 (Start)	0.9	0	1.7

3	Stop		

Time (minutes)	**Speed** (mph)	**Incline** (%)	**MET Level**
0 (Start)	0.9	0	1.7
2	1.0	0	1.8
4	Stop		

Time (minutes)	**Speed** (mph)	**Incline** (%)	**MET Level**
0 (Start)	1.0	0	1.8
2	1.1	0	1.85
4	Stop		

Time (minutes)	**Speed** (mph)	**Incline** (%)	**MET Level**
0 (Start)	1.0	0	1.8
2½	1.2	0	1.85
5	Stop		

Time (minutes)	**Speed** (mph)	**Incline** (%)	**MET Level**
0 (Start)	1.1	0	1.85
2½	1.3	.5	1.9
5	Stop		

Time (minutes)	**Speed** (mph)	**Incline** (%)	**MET Level**
0 (Start)	1.2	0	1.9

3	1.4	1	2.3
6	Stop		

Time (minutes)	**Speed** (mph)	**Incline** (%)	**MET Level**
0 (Start)	1.4	0	2.1
4	1.6	1	2.5
8	Stop		

Time (minutes)	**Speed** (mph)	**Incline** (%)	**MET Level**
0 (Start)	1.6	0	2.2
5	1.8	1	2.6
10	Stop		

Time (minutes)	**Speed** (mph)	**Incline** (%)	**MET Level**
0 (Start)	1.6	0	2.2
5	1.8	1	2.6
10	Cool-Down		
12½	Stop		

Moderate Intensity Protocols (3.0-5.9 METs)

Time (minutes)	**Speed** (mph)	**Incline** (%)	**MET Level**
0 (Start)	1.6	0	2.2
5	1.8	1	2.6
10	2.0	2	3.1
12½	Cool-Down		
15	Stop		

Time (minutes)	**Speed** (mph)	**Incline** (%)	**MET Level**
0 (Start)	1.6	0	2.2
5	1.8	1	2.6
10	2.0	2	3.1
15	Cool-Down		
17½	Stop		

Time (minutes)	**Speed** (mph)	**Incline** (%)	**MET Level**
0 (Start)	1.6	0	2.2
5	1.8	1	2.6
10	2.0	2	3.1
15	2.2	3	3.6
17½	Cool-Down		
20	Stop		

Time (minutes)	**Speed** (mph)	**Incline** (%)	**MET Level**
0 (Start)	1.8	1	2.6
5	2.0	2	3.1
10	2.2	3	3.6
15	2.4	4	4.2
17½	Cool-Down		
20	Stop		

Time (minutes)	**Speed** (mph)	**Incline** (%)	**MET Level**
0 (Start)	1.9	2	3.0
5	2.1	3	2.9
10	2.3	4	3.7
15	2.5	5	4.7
17½	Cool-Down		
20	Stop		

Time (minutes)	**Speed** (mph)	**Incline** (%)	**MET Level**
0 (Start)	2.0	0	2.5
5	2.2	2	3.3
10	2.4	4	4.2
15	2.6	6	5.1
17½	Cool-Down		
20	Stop		

Time (minutes)	**Speed** (mph)	**Incline** (%)	**MET Level**
0 (Start)	2.1	1	2.9
5	2.3	3	3.7
10	2.5	5	4.7
15	2.7	7	5.7
17½	Cool-Down		
20	Stop		

High Intensity Protocols (≥6.0 METs)

Time (minutes)	**Speed** (mph)	**Incline** (%)	**MET Level**
0 (Start)	2.2	2	3.3
5	2.4	4	4.2
10	2.6	6	5.1
15	2.8	8	6.2
17½	Cool-Down		
20	Stop		

Time (minutes)	**Speed** (mph)	**Incline** (%)	**MET Level**
0 (Start)	2.3	3	3.7
5	2.5	5	4.7
10	2.7	7	5.7
15	2.9	9	6.8

17½	Cool-Down		
20	Stop		

Time (minutes)	**Speed** (mph)	**Incline** (%)	**MET Level**
0 (Start)	2.1	1	2.9
5	2.4	4	4.2
10	2.7	7	5.7
15	3.0	10	7.4
17½	Cool-Down		
20	Stop		

Time (minutes)	**Speed** (mph)	**Incline** (%)	**MET Level**
0 (Start)	2.2	2	3.3
5	2.5	5	4.7
10	2.8	8	6.2
15	3.1	11	8.1
17½	Cool-Down		
20	Stop		

Time (minutes)	**Speed** (mph)	**Incline** (%)	**MET Level**
0 (Start)	2.3	3	3.7
5	2.6	6	5.1
10	2.9	9	6.8

15	3.2	12	8.8
17½	Cool-Down		
20	Stop		

Time (minutes)	**Speed** (mph)	**Incline** (%)	**MET Level**
0 (Start)	2.4	4	4.2
5	2.7	7	5.7
10	3.0	10	7.4
15	3.3	13	9.5
17½	Cool-Down		
20	Stop		

Time (minutes)	**Speed** (mph)	**Incline** (%)	**MET Level**
0 (Start)	2.5	5	4.7
5	2.8	8	6.2
10	3.1	11	8.1
15	3.4	14	10.2
17½	Cool-Down		
20	Stop		

Time (minutes)	**Speed** (mph)	**Incline** (%)	**MET Level**
0 (Start)	2.6	6	5.1
5	2.9	9	6.8

10	3.2	12	8.8
15	3.5	15	10.9
17½	Cool-Down		
20	Stop		

Breaks: You will notice that these protocols start very gently for those that are new to exercise or more debilitated and gradually increase in intensity. You will also notice that once a patient reaches a certain intensity, we build a rest period of lower intensity walking into the protocol to give the them a chance to catch their breath, lower their heart rate and blood pressure and increase their oxygen saturation before going up again to the peak.

Treadmill Protocols with Breaks

Time (minutes)	**Speed** (mph)	**Incline** (%)	**MET Level**
0 (Start)	1.6	0	2.2
5	1.8	1	2.6
10	2.0	2	3.1
13	1.5	0	2.15
16	2.2	3	3.6
18½	Cool-Down		
20	Stop		

Time (minutes)	**Speed** (mph)	**Incline** (%)	**MET Level**
0 (Start)	1.8	1	2.6
5	2.0	2	3.1
10	2.2	3	3.6
13	1.7	0	2.3
16	2.4	4	4.2
18½	Cool-Down		
20	Stop		

Time (minutes)	**Speed** (mph)	**Incline** (%)	**MET Level**
0 (Start)	1.9	2	3.0
5	2.1	3	2.9
10	2.3	4	3.7
13	1.8	1	2.6
16	2.5	5	4.7
18½	Cool-Down		
20	Stop		

Time (minutes)	**Speed** (mph)	**Incline** (%)	**MET Level**
0 (Start)	2.0	0	2.5
5	2.2	2	3.3
10	2.4	4	4.2
13	1.9	0	2.45

16	2.6	6	5.1
18½	Cool-Down		
20	Stop		

Time (minutes)	**Speed** (mph)	**Incline** (%)	**MET Level**
0 (Start)	2.1	1	2.9
5	2.3	3	3.7
10	2.5	5	4.7
13	2.0	0	2.5
16	2.7	7	5.7
18½	Cool-Down		
20	Stop		

Time (minutes)	**Speed** (mph)	**Incline** (%)	**MET Level**
0 (Start)	2.2	2	3.3
5	2.4	4	4.2
10	2.6	6	5.1
13	2.1	1	2.9
16	2.8	8	6.2
18½	Cool-Down		
20	Stop		

Time (minutes)	**Speed** (mph)	**Incline** (%)	**MET Level**
0 (Start)	2.3	3	3.7
5	2.5	5	4.7
10	2.7	7	5.7
13	2.2	2	3.3
16	2.9	9	6.8
18½	Cool-Down		
20	Stop		

Time (minutes)	**Speed** (mph)	**Incline** (%)	**MET Level**
0 (Start)	2.1	1	2.9
5	2.4	4	4.2
10	2.7	7	5.7
13	2.0	0	2.5
18	3.0	10	7.4
20½	Cool-Down		
23	Stop		

Time (minutes)	**Speed** (mph)	**Incline** (%)	**MET Level**
0 (Start)	2.2	2	3.3
5	2.5	5	4.7
10	2.8	8	6.2

13	2.1	1	2.9
18	3.1	11	8.1
20½	Cool-Down		
23	Stop		

Time (minutes)	**Speed** (mph)	**Incline** (%)	**MET Level**
0 (Start)	2.3	3	3.7
5	2.6	6	5.1
10	2.9	9	6.8
13	2.2	2	3.3
18	3.2	12	8.8
20½	Cool-Down		
23	Stop		

Time (minutes)	**Speed** (mph)	**Incline** (%)	**MET Level**
0 (Start)	2.4	4	4.2
5	2.7	7	5.7
10	3.0	10	7.4
13	2.3	3	3.7
18	3.3	13	9.5
20½	Cool-Down		
23	Stop		

Time (minutes)	**Speed** (mph)	**Incline** (%)	**MET Level**
0 (Start)	2.5	5	4.7
5	2.8	8	6.2
10	3.1	11	8.1
13	2.4	4	4.2
18	3.4	14	10.2
20½	Cool-Down		
23	Stop		

Time (minutes)	**Speed** (mph)	**Incline** (%)	**MET Level**
0 (Start)	2.6	6	5.1
5	2.9	9	6.8
10	3.2	12	8.8
13	2.5	5	4.7
18	3.5	15	10.9
20½	Cool-Down		
23	Stop		

CHAPTER 9
NUTRITION

"The doctor of the future will no longer treat the human frame with drugs, but rather will cure and prevent disease with nutrition."
– Thomas Edison

Written with gratitude to my Co-Author, Meredith Liss, MA, RDN, CDN, CDE, CLT

The subject of nutrition will almost invariably be included in any meaningful discussion of health and wellness. In the context of living well with a pulmonary disease, the conversation should be at least slightly (and in many cases, vastly) different than what most of us are used to hearing (and eating). In fact, sometimes recommendations made for the general population, particularly as they relate to cardiovascular diseases, diabetes, and obesity can actually be in direct conflict with the needs of people living with respiratory conditions.

Before I begin, please understand that this chapter is not a substitute for the medical advice of your physician or a personal consultation with a nutritionist. Instead this chapter is a compilation of what I have come to believe are the most important principles as they relate to eating (and living) well with a pulmonary disease as well as information that will have the greatest impact on your respiratory system in particular as well as your overall pulmonary wellness.

I'll begin by telling you a story to illustrate many of the issues regarding nutrition in the context of living with pulmonary disease. Perhaps you know this story. It's one that patients have been telling me for years and one that I've heard at least a hundred (if not a thousand) times before.

Last night, my wife (or husband or any other person) and I went out for dinner at our favorite Italian (or any other favorite) restaurant. When we left the house, my breathing was fine, and I was able to walk the five blocks to the restaurant. I had to stop once or twice to catch my breath, but I was able to do it.

We had a wonderful time. After dinner, though, I was really having difficulty breathing. In fact, after about a block and a half, I was so short of breath that we had to take a taxi the rest of the way home. I don't understand what happened.

Well, I understand completely, and it's more common than you might think. When someone tells me this story, I have a pretty standard line of questioning that goes something like this:

Me: Did you have an appetizer?

Patient: Yes. Shrimp cocktail.

Me: I see. Anything else?

Patient: Yes. We shared an order of calamari.

Me: Right. Was the calamari fried?

Patient: Is there any other kind?

Me: I'll ask the questions. Was there bread on the table?

Patient: It's an Italian restaurant. Of course there was bread.

Me: How many pieces did you have?

Patient: Two, maybe three.

Me: Butter?

Patient: Olive oil.

Me: What did you have for your main course?

Patient: Chicken Parmesan.

Me: Sounds delicious. Pasta too?

Patient: Linguini.

Me: What kind of sauce?

Patient: Tomato.

Me: Dessert?

Patient: Tiramisu.

Me: Alcohol?

Patient: Two Scotch and Sodas.

Me: Coffee?

Patient: Cappuccino.

Me: How did you sleep?

Patient: Terrible! I was up the whole night.

Me: Really? Why is that?

Patient: First, I had terrible reflux.

Me: Then?

Patient: I was coughing all night.

Me: And how do you feel today?

Patient: Exhausted.

Me: Anything else?

Patient: Yeah. I'm very dry.

Me: Anything else?

Patient: Yeah. I'm constipated.

Sound familiar?

Like breathing itself, eating and nutrition are multi-factorial processes. The dynamics involved in what, why, and how people eat are many, diverse, and individualized; from physical and physiological, to intellectual, educational and emotional, to financial and logistical, among many other factors.

As a result, we must first consider the impact that food has on breathing so you can begin to eat intelligently, systematically *and* in a manner that reasonably fits your lifestyle because if it doesn't, you *probably* won't do it and you *definitely* won't be able to sustain it; in which case, these recommendations *definitely* won't work. These strategies include thinking about and planning what happens before, during, and after individual meals, over the course of a given day or week *and* the weeks, months, or years to come.

Also like breathing, the process of eating and nutrition can be divided into both mechanical and chemical processes. Therefore, I think it will be useful for you to have a basic understanding of the anatomy of the digestive system, particularly as it relates to the mechanics of breathing as well as the classifications of foods and their nutrients as they relate to our body's chemistry. By understanding these concepts, you'll be able to organize your eating behaviors to maximize your respiratory health and overall wellbeing.

I would bet that the overwhelming majority of people have a general (if not specific) idea of which foods are healthy and which foods are not, which foods will cause us to gain weight and which ones will help us lose weight; and which foods we should eat and which ones we should avoid, as well as which ones we should throw right in the trash.

Despite this basic knowledge, diet and nutrition remains one of the most difficult areas for people to implement and maintain successful and lasting changes in their lives. In the context of pulmonary disease, we also have the added responsibility of thinking about which foods (and other eating behaviors) will make us more or less short of breath.

Nutrition is an extremely important, yet not extremely well understood component of living well with a pulmonary disease. While there is a tremendous wealth of knowledge about nutrition in the management of conditions like cardiovascular disease, diabetes, and obesity; far less is understood about the role of nutrition as it relates specifically to pulmonary health and wellness. This is particularly problematic because the *what, when, why, and how we eat* all exert a tremendous impact on our health in general and our respiratory health and wellbeing in particular.

As you probably know by now, I am completely biased in favor of exercise as the single greatest behavioral change you can implement to improve your health. However, nutrition comes in a very close second. In many cases (e.g. someone who is either severely overweight or severely underweight: two common scenarios in pulmonary disease), nutrition can even take center stage as your most important health priority.

Some nutritional issues will have a direct impact on our breathing. Some will be felt immediately, such as the increase in shortness of breath that you might experience after consuming a large meal (or a carbonated beverage or alcohol). Others will have more of an indirect or incidental effect, occurring over a longer period of time, such as the increased work of breathing that occurs following a 25-pound winter weight gain.

Conversely, not only do eating and nutrition impact your breathing, but breathing can also affect eating and nutrition. For example, being overweight, particularly around the midsection, can increase your shortness of breath. Now, with each breath, your body has to lift those extra pounds around your waist. This can make activity more difficult, causing you to become more sedentary. As a result of this sedentary lifestyle, your body will burn fewer calories, causing you to gain even more weight (or at least making the weight more difficult to lose).

As another example, shortness of breath can decrease your appetite or impair your ability to prepare meals, making it a challenge to consume an adequate number of calories. Additionally, many people with respiratory disease are hyper-metabolic, meaning that they burn many times the normal amount of calories than the average person. This accelerated metabolism is due to increased frequency (think respiratory rate) and work (think effort or intensity) of breathing.

As you can see, the processes of respiration and eating are intimately related and like many of the other cycles we have talked about, these processes can either work for or against you. My goal is to eliminate some of the mystery behind these relationships and improve your understanding of how you can best help yourself and your body get the most *out* of what you put *in.*

Steve Covey, author of *The Seven Habits of Highly Effective People*, has a great quote: "the main thing is to keep the main thing the main thing." As healthcare professionals, it is imperative for clinicians to spend an adequate amount of time learning about their patients. This includes understanding both the medical aspects of their disease, as well as getting to know them as human beings. We need to find out about their families, occupations and personal habits (including what they eat) so we can ensure our patients' main thing remains the main thing.

As one example, in the context of Ultimate Pulmonary Wellness, many people don't get enough exercise. Others may be taking their medications incorrectly. For others, anxiety or depression may be their most paralyzing limitation. However, for many of our patients, nutrition is by far, their greatest challenge.

By meticulously getting to know each patient, we can focus on their most important priorities and not waste time on circumstances that do not apply to them. That being said, in most people's situations, nutrition should definitely be included as one of the top priorities.

Basic Anatomy and Physiology of the Digestive System

The process of digestion begins in the mouth, where mastication (a fancy word for chewing) begins to *mechanically* break down food into smaller pieces. At the same time, enzymes in your saliva begin to *chemically* break down starches into simple sugars. From the mouth, food passes through the esophagus, which moves it into the stomach through a series of muscular contractions called *peristalsis.*

This step is very important and can often have a major impact on the respiratory system. The esophagus sits just behind the trachea, where the *epiglottis* prevents food from entering the trachea during swallowing. However, if the epiglottis is not functioning properly, food and other digestive contents (including stomach acid) can enter the trachea or even the smaller airways and the lungs.

When foreign materials enter the respiratory tract, they can trigger inflammation or obstruction in the pharynx, larynx, trachea, airways, and lungs. For a person who already has trouble breathing, this *reflux* can compound their respiratory problem by causing bronchoconstriction (or bronchospasm), increased mucus production or aspiration, when food or other substances are breathed directly into the airways or lungs, potentially leading to inflammation and/or infection.

From the esophagus, food travels through the lower esophageal sphincter into the stomach. The stomach is a hollow organ that churns the food with digestive enzymes and stomach acid. Food is further broken down into smaller and smaller particles and proteins are broken down into their component building blocks, amino acids.

From the stomach, food moves into the small intestine, which is made up of three parts: the duodenum, jejunum, and ileum. In the duodenum, food mixes with bile from the gallbladder (produced by the liver), neutralizing stomach acid and aiding in the digestion of fats. Enzymes from the pancreas also assist in the digestion of proteins, carbohydrates, and complex sugars. Nutrients are absorbed as they pass through the jejunum and ileum, including glucose (sugar), fatty acids, vitamins, and minerals. From the small intestine, waste products pass into the colon (large intestine), where water and minerals are reabsorbed into the blood, producing solid stool (debris and bacteria) for elimination through the rectum and anus.

The Relationship Between Eating and Breathing

Now, let's introduce a concept that is crucial to your understanding of how to maximize your nutritional status: the relationship between food, eating, digestion—and breathing. As I mentioned previously, some of these issues will directly impact your breathing, whereas others will have a more indirect effect. Some of these factors will be interconnected, and others will be stand-alone issues.

As I see it, the primary issues related to nutrition (food, eating, and digestion); as they affect and are affected by respiratory disease; can be broken down into several major categories. I will address each of them, one by one, and it will be up to you and your healthcare team to decide which issues are most important for you, and which ones may not apply to you at all.

Mechanical Aspects of Eating and Breathing

For the purposes of this discussion, it will be helpful if you think of the upper body as being divided into two separate compartments, similar to a suitcase. The upper compartment, called the thorax or thoracic cavity, houses the heart (within the mediastinum) and the lungs. The lower compartment, called the abdomen or abdominal cavity contains the stomach, liver, gallbladder, spleen, pancreas, intestines, kidneys, and adrenal glands. These two cavities are divided by the dome-shaped diaphragm; the primary muscle of inspiration.

The thoracic and abdominal cavities each have their own internal pressures called intra-thoracic and intra-abdominal pressures, respectively. However, even though they are separate entities, the intra-thoracic and intra-abdominal pressures are intimately related and can directly influence each other. If the pressure in one cavity rises, pressure in the other cavity can also rise (and vice versa).

Again, let's think back to our suitcase analogy with one side of the suitcase being the thorax and the other side, the abdomen. If you overstuff the thoracic side (as in the case of Emphysema)—the hyper-inflated (overfilled) lungs push downward, compressing the diaphragm and abdominal contents, increasing the pressure on the abdominal side. If you overstuff the abdominal side (as in the case of a large meal or constipation or bloating), the abdominal contents will push upward, resisting diaphragmatic excursion and lung expansion, increasing the pressure on the thoracic side.

Now, here's where things get interesting. The dome-shaped diaphragm lies between the thorax and the abdomen, sitting directly below the lungs in the thorax and above the stomach and intestines in the abdomen. When you take a breath, the diaphragm contracts in a downward direction, creating a negative pressure in the thorax. This negative pressure is what causes air to rush in, filling the lungs.

When the pressure in the abdominal cavity is increased (e.g. after you've eaten a large meal or become bloated with gas), there is increased resistance against the diaphragm's downward contraction. This puts the diaphragm at a significant mechanical disadvantage, making diaphragmatic contraction more difficult and causing you to feel more short of breath.

In addition, the lungs can get pushed upwards and compressed, further reducing the amount of air that can be taken in with each breath. In an effort to make up for this reduced *volume* of air, you're now forced to breathe faster and more shallowly, working harder for each breath. If you recall from previous chapters, the more forcefully you try to breathe, the more airway narrowing, alveolar collapse and air trapping occurs, further increasing your work of breathing and shortness of breath.

Now, here is some further food for thought (pun intended). It doesn't matter if the obstruction is solid, liquid, or gas: full is full. This means that you have to pay attention to the amount of solid food you ingest, the amount of liquid that you drink and the amount of gas you ingest (or produce). One way that this can occur is by accidentally swallowing air when you eat. However, if fullness and bloating are an issue for you, you should consider limiting carbonated beverages as well as solid foods and liquids known to cause gas.

Chemical Aspects of Eating and Breathing

It is important to realize that not all foods are created equal with respect to their chemical impact on breathing. Each type of food carries a specific chemical load. In particular, it is essential to realize that gram for gram; carbohydrate metabolism produces more carbon dioxide (CO_2) than the metabolism of either protein or fat. This is what makes high-carbohydrate meals particularly challenging for people with lung disease. Depending upon the size of the meal, the amount of carbohydrates, and the severity of your disease, results can vary from mild discomfort to acute respiratory distress.

The *Respiratory Quotient* (RQ) or *Respiratory Coefficient* is the ratio between the amount of carbon dioxide produced by the body and the amount of oxygen consumed during the metabolism of food. Carbohydrates have an RQ of 1.0. Proteins have an RQ of 0.8, and fat has an RQ of 0.7. In other words, if you eat 1 gram of protein, its RQ of 0.8 would produce only 80% of the carbon dioxide that would be produced by 1 gram of carbohydrate. If you eat 1 gram of fat, its RQ of 0.7 would produce only 70% of the carbon dioxide that would be produced by 1 gram of carbohydrate. In other words, eating a high carbohydrate meal can place a substantially greater workload on the respiratory system due to increased levels of CO_2 in the blood.

So, with every strand of spaghetti you eat (slight exaggeration), chemical receptors send a message to your brain that the CO_2 level in your blood is high, which, as you may recall, is one of the primary stimuli of respiration. When the CO_2 level in your blood rises, the brain sends out chemical impulses telling your respiratory system to breathe faster, deeper, and more forcefully, further increasing the work of breathing *and your SOB.*

Metabolism: Food as Fuel

Metabolism is a set of life-sustaining chemical processes and reactions that take place in every cell of our bodies. These include the process of digestion—the breaking down of foods into their component nutrients to release and supply energy and other essential substances to sustain all bodily structures and functions.

In the same way that a car needs to refuel every certain number of miles, we continually need to provide our bodies with the necessary nutrients based on the metabolic demands of our daily activities and individual energy use. At the most basic level, we eat in order to provide energy for our bodies to carry out all of the functions of metabolism.

Nutritional Value of Foods

Besides the mechanical impact of food on breathing, it is also important to realize that not all foods are created equal. From a *nutritional* perspective, it may help to expand on our automobile analogy. In the same way that there are different grades of gasoline that can either enhance or hinder your vehicle's performance, the foods we eat can similarly affect our functioning. The higher the *quality* of the nutrients (food) we provide, the more efficiently they can be used and the higher "performance" you can expect from your body in the form of increased energy and activity tolerance and ultimately, reduced SOB.

What Should We Eat?

The *Harvard School of Public Health* created the *Healthy Eating Plate and the Healthy Eating Pyramid*. Instead of focusing only on the *quantity* we eat, Harvard's *Healthy Eating Plate* places equal—if not more—emphasis on food *quality*. In addition, the Healthy Eating Pyramid includes daily exercise and weight control in its core principles, two areas of particular importance for people living with a pulmonary disease.

According to the Harvard group, half of your plate should be made up of fruits and vegetables. A quarter of your plate should be made up of *whole* grains (not just any grains), and the remaining quarter of your plate should be *healthy* protein. They also recommend using *healthy* fats and oils and drinking plenty of water as well as coffee or tea, with no more than 1 to 2 servings of milk and dairy per day.

Please keep in mind that like everything else we discuss, there are caveats and exceptions to all recommendations or suggestions in this text and individual conditions must be applied. Many factors will determine what and how you should eat, including your age, gender, activity level, medical conditions(s), and medication(s). For this reason, rather than give you exact recommendations regarding specific foods and amounts, I'll present some general principles, which you can further explore with your physician, nutritionist, and other members of your healthcare team. Here is a link to the Harvard HEP:

http://www.hsph.harvard.edu/nutritionsource/healthy-eating-plate

Fruits and Vegetables (½ Plate)

Fruits and vegetables are high in many essential nutrients and low in fat, sodium, and calories. They also have zero cholesterol. Eating a diet rich in fruits and vegetables is associated with improved pulmonary function and reduced risk of cardiovascular disease (e.g. hypertension, heart attack, and stroke), obesity, type 2 diabetes, osteoporosis and may also protect against certain types of cancers. Fruits and vegetables are also high in fiber, which lowers cholesterol and promotes healthy bowel function. No single fruit or vegetable contains all of the nutrients that you need, so try to eat a wide variety to maximize your nutritional benefit.

Although Harvard's system suggests a combination of fruits and vegetables to comprise half of your plate, it is preferable—particularly for pulmonary patients—to focus on *non-starchy* (i.e. low-carb) vegetables, while grouping *starchy* (i.e. high-carb) vegetables with the grain portion of the plate.

Non-starchy vegetables include (but are not limited to) green leafy vegetables such as arugula, kale, spinach, Swiss chard and watercress, as well as artichokes, asparagus, broccoli, Brussels sprouts, carrots, cauliflower, celery, cucumbers, eggplant, garlic, jicama, leeks, mushrooms, okra, onions, peppers, radishes, red cabbage, scallions, snow peas, tomatoes, yellow squash, and zucchini. Many of these can be eaten raw or cooked.

When we are talking about fruit, we mean fresh or frozen fruit, *not* juice or dried fruit as these are highly concentrated in carbs (sugars) and therefore, should be limited to two to three servings per day. Here are a few examples of a fruit serving: a small apple, ½ medium banana, ¾ cup of blackberries, ¾ cup of blueberries, 15 grapes, ½ mango, 1 cup of melon, small orange, peach, pear, ¾ cup of pineapple, 2 small plums, 1 cup of raspberries, and 1¼ cup of strawberries. The greater the variety you include, the healthier. Again, include but do not exceed two to three servings per day.

Whole Grains (¼ Plate)

Grains can be divided into whole grains and refined or processed grains. Whole grains contain the entire grain kernel (bran, germ, and endosperm) plus dietary fiber. Refined grains have been milled to remove the bran and germ, giving a finer texture and prolonging their shelf life. However, the refining process also removes the dietary fiber, iron and many B vitamins—in other words, most of the good stuff.

Whole grains are high in many essential nutrients, including dietary fiber, B vitamins (thiamin, riboflavin, niacin, and folic acid) and minerals (iron, magnesium, and selenium). Eating a diet rich in whole grains can lower cholesterol, reducing the risk of cardiovascular disease, stabilizing blood sugar and lowering the risk of type 2 diabetes and obesity. A diet high in fiber also promotes healthy bowel function and can help prevent blood clots, a known cause of heart attack and stroke. Whenever possible, choose whole grains and whole grain products over processed grains for maximum nutritional benefit.

Whole grains include whole wheat (bread, cereal, or pasta), rye, barley and bulgur, as well as gluten-free whole grains like buckwheat, millet, steel-cut oats, quinoa and brown rice. Many products are made from refined grains including white flour, white bread and white rice. "Enriched" grains have some of the B vitamins (thiamin, riboflavin, niacin, and folic acid) and iron added back but they are still not as healthy as whole grains.

When designating a quarter of your plate for whole grains, pulmonary patients should choose *either* a portion of whole grains *or* a portion of starchy vegetables, *not both*. For example, brown rice *or* whole-wheat pasta *or* potatoes *or* corn and *not* all of the above.

Healthy Protein (¼ Plate)

Protein can be obtained from both animal and plant sources and is crucial in the composition of bones, muscles, cartilage, skin, hair, and blood as well as enzymes, hormones and vitamins, particularly the B vitamins. Proteins are also high in iron, which is critical in the transport of oxygen in the blood; magnesium, which is essential for building bones and releasing energy from the muscles; and zinc, which is important for fueling many biochemical reactions and boosting immune function.

While protein is essential for a healthy diet, some high-protein foods are healthier than others, so choose your protein sources wisely. Many foods that are high in protein (particularly protein from animal sources) also contain high amounts of sodium and/or saturated (unhealthy) fats. For example, although high in protein, red meat can contain high levels of both sodium and saturated fat. Processed meats (e.g. bacon, sausage, cold cuts) are notorious for being high in sodium and other chemicals often associated with inflammation and chronic diseases.

Therefore, it's preferable to choose healthy proteins like organic grass-fed beef (which is lower in saturated fat than conventional grain-fed beef), organic eggs, organic skinless poultry and wild-caught fish; and limiting processed meat products.

When it comes to fish, be sure to include at least two meals per week of cold-water fatty fish such as salmon, sardines, herring, or mackerel for the anti-inflammatory benefit of the omega-3 fatty acids. You can also obtain protein from non-animal sources such as legumes (e.g. chickpeas, black beans, lentils), tofu, tempeh, seitan, unsalted nuts or seeds, and nut butters (e.g. peanut, cashew, almond).

Healthy Fats and Oils

Although fats and oils are often viewed as the enemy—leading to obesity, heart disease and a host of other health problems—this is not the case. In fact, healthy fats are cardio-*protective*, meaning that they actually protect the heart from atherosclerosis and coronary disease. Due to their high calorie content, healthy oils are particularly beneficial for patients who have a difficult time gaining or maintaining weight.

Fats can be classified into four main categories: saturated fat, polyunsaturated fat, monounsaturated fat, and trans-fat or trans-fatty acids.

Saturated fat can raise your blood cholesterol, a known risk factor for heart disease. Therefore, you definitely want to limit the amount of saturated fat in your diet by eating less butter, high-fat cheeses, poultry skin, conventional grain-fed beef and any products made with palm kernel oil.

Polyunsaturated fats include both omega-6 fatty acids and omega-3 fatty acids. Both are essential for our diet. However, it is important to maintain the correct ratio of omega-6 fats to omega-3 fats. The American diet contains excess omega-6 fatty acids because so many processed foods are made with vegetable oils derived from corn, cottonseed, safflower, sunflower, soybean, and "mixed vegetable oils."

We still need them in our diet, but when consumed *in excess*, omega-6 fats can trigger or increase inflammation. While this can be beneficial in times of illness or injury, inflammation is associated with increased risk of heart disease, diabetes, arthritis, osteoporosis, cancer, and respiratory disease. For all of these reasons, it is recommended that we increase our intake of anti-inflammatory omega-3 fatty acids while limiting our intake of pro-inflammatory omega-6 fatty acids.

As I mentioned, the main sources of omega-3 fatty acids are cold-water fatty fish such as salmon, sardines, herring, or mackerel. If you are not a fish lover, you can get your omega-3 fats from land sources such as walnuts, ground flaxseeds, chia seeds, hemp seeds, canola oil and green leafy vegetables. You can also consider taking a supplement, which will be addressed later in this chapter.

When it comes to fats and oils, the bottom line is to enjoy foods rich in monounsaturated fats such as avocado, unsalted nuts and nut butters, seeds, olives and olive oil.

Finally, trans-fats or *trans-fatty acids* are man-made fats. However, as of June 15, 2015, they have been taken off the FDA's Safe List and should be avoided at all costs. Trans-fats can be found in foods like margarine, commercially fried foods and baked goods made with either shortening or partially hydrogenated vegetable oils.

Dairy and Bone Health

Dairy products are a good source of calcium, vitamin D and potassium, and yogurt is an excellent source of probiotics, which are beneficial to digestive health. My gut feeling (pun intended) is that probiotics and the overall health of our gut also play a key role in reducing inflammation and boosting our immune function. However, according to the Harvard group, while calcium is important for building and maintaining healthy bones, there may be other sources that may be healthier and lead to fewer associated health risks. If you do plan to use dairy, replace whole milk, yogurt, and cheese with low-fat or fat-free products and limit their use to a maximum of one to two servings per day.

If you take or have taken steroids, you may be at increased risk for bone loss (i.e. osteopenia and osteoporosis). Therefore, it is important to pay attention to your intake of calcium *and* vitamin D (which aids in calcium absorption) and magnesium (to prevent any negative side effects of calcium).

Calcium-rich foods include dark green, leafy vegetables, canned sardines with bones, canned salmon, black-eyed peas, yogurt, cow's milk, cheese, calcium-fortified nut milks, and firm tofu. Adults ages 19-50 require 1000 mg per day. When women turn 50 and men turn 70, the requirement increases to 1200 mg daily.

Foods rich in vitamin D include salmon, tuna, sardines, eggs, fortified milk, and yogurt. Magnesium-rich foods include spinach, black beans, pumpkin seeds, almonds, cashews, soymilk, peanut butter, avocado, whole grain bread, brown rice, yogurt, salmon and milk.

Dairy and Mucus Production

For as long as I can remember, people have been claiming that dairy products increase mucus production. I'm not going to make a case as to whether I think they do or don't. I will, however, remind you that everyone is different. So, if you feel that dairy products increase *your* mucus production, avoid them.

However, many people with COPD and other conditions in which mucus is a problem *are* able to tolerate at least some dairy. If you want to include dairy products in your diet, I wouldn't just accept the fact that you can't just because people have said so. This is particularly important for people who might be prone to calcium or vitamin D deficiency, including anyone who has been on steroids or who has additional protein needs due to muscle loss or weakness. Also, don't forget the probiotic benefits of yogurt for anyone who has taken antibiotics.

Not all dairy products are created equal. Most people find that skim products are easier to handle than whole dairy, but my suggestion would be to *try* them if you like them and see how you react (unless you are lactose intolerant or allergic). Also, start slow. Instead of drinking a quart of milk, try a sip or two or a couple of spoonfuls of yogurt. If you tolerate this amount, you can gradually increase your "dosage."

Maintaining a Healthy Weight

Keeping your body at a healthy weight is extremely important and should be included in any discussion regarding the optimal management of pulmonary disease and health in general. This includes maintaining a normal weight versus being either over- or underweight as well as promoting good body composition (the percentages and ratios of body fat, lean muscle, bone, and water). As you probably realize, not all body weight is created equal.

To many, it may seem like being overweight or underweight are simply equal but opposite problems. If you're overweight, you simply need to eat less and get your butt off the couch and if you're underweight, I'm sure at some point, you've had to suffer the indignity of someone telling you how "lucky" you are because "you can eat anything you want and not gain weight."

However, *simply* losing or gaining weight is not actually simple at all. In fact, it can be extremely complex, especially in the context of pulmonary disease. In addition, sometimes your ability to lose or gain weight can be completely unrelated to anything you eat or don't eat or any exercise you do or don't do.

For example, if you've ever had to take steroids, you know prednisone can cause you to gain weight, particularly around the face and midsection. And for those of you who spend a good amount of your day gasping for air, you already know what it feels like to run a marathon—every day! While being overweight can have a significantly negative impact on your respiratory mechanics and your disease, being underweight is often a negative *consequence* of your disease.

If you have pulmonary disease and have either tried to lose weight or gain weight, you probably know that doing either one requires a sound (scientific) plan and a very healthy dose of willpower. Wouldn't it be great if those who are overweight could simply "donate" those extra pounds to those that are underweight? Of course, the situation is not always this cut and dried but let me explain further.

The Overweight Patient

As I mentioned earlier, being overweight can have a profoundly negative impact on your respiratory mechanics and increase your work of breathing. However, depending on the amount of excess weight, the problem can range from being a minor annoyance (if you are five or ten pounds overweight) to literally being the difference between life and death. I often see patients who are 25, 50, or even 100+ pounds overweight. If you are more than 25 pounds overweight, weight loss is unquestionably your highest priority and without a concentrated effort to lose the weight, it will be virtually impossible for you to achieve your full potential.

In addition to *how much* excess weight you are carrying, *where* your weight sits on your body can also have a major impact on breathing. In particular, excess weight around the abdominal area will make breathing more difficult, forcing you to lift that excess weight with every breath. Think of it as weightlifting for your respiratory muscles. Is it any wonder why you're more fatigued?

Often, patients come to me with reports of increased shortness of breath even though their pulmonary function has remained stable. In fact, not much has changed at all except that they are now 15, 20, or 25 pounds heavier than the last time I saw them. Think of those extra pounds as two bowling balls pulling down on your thorax every time you need to take a breath. Being overweight contributes to increased shortness of breath, low energy and decreased activity tolerance. Often, if patients can manage to lose the extra weight, their breathing problems improve dramatically.

When it comes to losing weight, exercise alone will *not* do it. Exercise is a major part of weight loss but diet is at least equally if not more critical. In fact, I often tell my patients that they have the ability to out-eat any exercise program we give them. The healthiest strategies will include a combination of both healthier eating *and* increased physical activity.

The Underweight Patient

The underweight patient faces a completely different set of challenges. Due to increased work and frequency of breathing, the body's metabolic (and caloric) demand can increase dramatically. I don't believe the "10 times that of a normal person" that I've been hearing lately, but the difference in metabolism is significant compared to someone who is not constantly struggling to breathe. If weight loss progresses far enough and the person does not have sufficient fat stores, they will begin to burn muscle tissue for fuel. By the time the body reaches this point, the patient is often too weak to carry out even the simplest daily activities. Unfortunately, once you get to this point, their overall prognosis is poor if they cannot reverse this process.

Caloric Value of Food

From a *caloric* perspective, both protein and carbohydrates contain 4 calories per gram as compared to fats, which contain 9 calories per gram and alcohol contains 7 calories per gram. This makes calorie-dense (but healthy) fats a friend to the person trying to gain weight. *Do not* increase your alcohol intake as a weight-gain strategy unless you don't plan on getting much done. In addition to harming your liver, I'm sure you can see how this choice could lead to a whole host of other problems.

Now, let's take it one step further. A pound is made up of *approximately* 3500 calories. This means that in order to lose or gain one pound, you must either create a deficit of 3500 calories or a surplus of 3500 calories, respectively. In other words, if I consume 3500 fewer calories than I burn,

I can reasonably expect to lose one pound. Conversely, if I consume 3500 calories more than I burn, I can expect to gain one pound.

Therefore, if your goal were to *lose* one pound per week, you'd need to create an average deficit of 500 calories per day (7 days per week x 500 calories per day = 3500 total calories). If your goal were to lose two pounds per week, you would need to create an average deficit of 1000 calories per day (7 x 1000 = 7000). This can be accomplished either by burning extra calories by increasing your exercise or activity, or by reducing your caloric intake by eating smaller portions or less calorie-dense foods. As I mentioned previously, a combination of both is more effective than either strategy alone.

Conversely, if your goal were to *gain* one pound per week, you'd need to create an average surplus of 500 calories per day. If your goal were to gain two pounds per week, you'd need to create an average surplus of 1000 calories per day. In the case of pulmonary patients, decreasing your activity is *not* recommended *at all.* Neither is increasing the size of your individual meals (which may not even be possible).

For all of these reasons, gaining weight is often even more challenging for the underweight person than losing weight is for the overweight person. If you are underweight, it is crucial that you utilize strategies to increase your caloric intake by eating as much calorie-dense (but still healthy) food as you can in a way that will not significantly impair your breathing.

Many factors contribute to weight changes and there are no absolutes. So, instead of thinking of this as a hard and fast rule, use this mathematical approach to calories as a rough *guideline.* Make any necessary adjustments based on your own individual experiences and the recommendations of your healthcare team.

Hydration and Fluid Balance

Maintaining adequate hydration is important for everyone, but it is particularly crucial for people with pulmonary disease. Firstly, every part of the respiratory tract requires moisture to do its job effectively. In addition, hydration is important for thinning out your secretions, (mucus) keeping it moist, and allowing it to be expelled more easily. When we are dehydrated, our mucus becomes thicker and stickier, making it more difficult to expel and making you more prone to infection.

Many people have difficulty getting adequate hydration during the day for a variety of reasons. These can include anything from "I don't like water" to "the more I drink, the more I pee," among others. If you are not naturally a big water drinker, I know you're not going to go from drinking zero glasses of water to drinking the "recommended" 8-10 glasses per day. However, try to aim for a minimum of 4-5 glasses per day. A good indicator that you are getting enough fluids is that your urine is clear and colorless. People who are dehydrated often have highly concentrated, dark yellow or cloudy urine.

Also, when we talk about getting enough fluids, other drinks besides water count toward your overall fluid goal. In fact, if you are trying to gain weight, you should *avoid* drinking a lot of water since it fills you up *without* the benefit of having any calories. Instead, opt for calorie-containing beverages such as non-fat milk, a smoothie or low or zero-carb protein drink to maximize your caloric intake without increasing your carbohydrate load.

Also, don't drink before or during your meals. This can fill you up and prevent you from getting adequate calories and nutrition from your food. If lack of appetite or a feeling of fullness is an issue, you can get some of your fluids in the form of fruits, vegetables, and soups. Just be careful though, because many soups contain a lot of sodium.

Conversely, people who are trying to lose weight should opt *only* for plain water or other non-caloric beverages whenever possible. You would be amazed at how many extra calories can be consumed in the form of caloric beverages. In addition, drinking water before or during a meal will make you feel more full, allowing you to eat less and reducing your overall caloric intake.

IMPORTANT: Some people have to be careful about consuming *too much* water. This includes people with renal (kidney) disease, heart failure and those taking diuretics, among others. While it is still important for these patients to remain hydrated, they should discuss their particular fluid requirements and restrictions with their physician.

Alcohol

When it comes to alcohol and cardiopulmonary disease, there are several considerations for you to be aware of. First, alcohol is a mild diuretic and increases the production of urine, making you pee more frequently. It also has a negative fluid impact, meaning if you drink one cup of alcohol, you lose more than one cup of fluid. Therefore, if you are going to drink alcohol, make sure that you are drinking extra (non-alcoholic) fluids to replace those flushed from your body to avoid becoming dehydrated (or too drunk).

Alcohol is a central nervous system depressant that lowers your heart rate and makes you breathe slower and more shallowly. Therefore, depending upon the condition of your lungs (and how much you drink), alcohol can make breathing more difficult, even causing respiratory distress or failure.

Also, alcohol can interact with your medications including prescription drugs, over the counter (OTC) drugs and nutritional supplements, potentially increasing the effects of some and making others less effective or not effective at all. Again, if you are going to drink alcohol, check with your doctor to determine if and how much is safe for you.

Finally, men and women metabolize alcohol differently. As a general rule, men should limit alcohol to a *maximum* of two drinks per day, and women should consume no more than one drink per day. Now, before you start looking for that 64-ounce beer mug from college, one drink means 5 ounces of wine, 12 ounces of beer, or 1½ ounces of liquor. (Sorry, sports fans.)

Please understand that I am not trying to scare you, nor am I trying to convince you to become a teetotaler. I'm not. All I am saying is to use common sense. Be aware of the effects of alcohol on your body, and if you do decide to drink, moderation is the key.

Caffeine

Caffeine is a central nervous system *stimulant*, potentially increasing your heart rate, blood pressure and respiratory rate. This is particularly important for pulmonary patients because their hearts are often already working harder due to the increased work of breathing. In addition, certain classes of pulmonary medications—*beta-2 agonists* in particular, can also be stimulants. Therefore, when used in combination, the two can make you feel jittery, anxious or shorter of breath in addition to difficulty sleeping. Stimulants can also increase your risk of cardiac arrhythmias like tachycardia (fast heart rate) or atrial fibrillation, among others.

Sodium (Salt)

Unrefined salt provides two elements essential for life, sodium and chloride. The American Heart Association recommends 1500 milligrams of sodium (or less) per day. However, while sodium is an essential nutrient, the average American often consumes more than double that amount and although seemingly harmless, most people don't understand the potential danger of an over-intake of salt.

Think back to our early discussions about the body maintaining equilibrium. This is true of the body's salinity (sodium level) as well. If you eat too much salt, your body will retain additional fluid to dilute the amount of sodium in your blood. This increased fluid retention can lead to an increase in blood pressure, causing the heart (particularly the left ventricle) to work harder. If left untreated over time, the ventricle can increase in overall size and thickness, requiring more oxygen to supply its increased muscle mass.

If the left ventricle cannot meet this excess demand (overload), fluid can back up into the pulmonary circulation, causing increased shortness of breath. This is known as left-sided or congestive heart failure. Left unchecked, blood can continue backwards through the pulmonary circulation to the right side of the heart, eventually pooling in the lower extremities (pedal edema). This is what is known as right-sided heart failure. The bottom line is "easy on the salt!"

Instead of salt, use onions, garlic, herbs, spices, citrus juices, and vinegars to flavor your food. Experiment with basil, curry, dill, oregano, paprika, parsley, rosemary, sage, thyme, turmeric and other salt-free flavorings.

Minimize your use of high sodium foods such as smoked, cured, salted, or canned meat, fish or poultry (including bacon, cold cuts, ham, hot dogs, sausage, caviar and anchovies). Opt for fresh or frozen vegetables instead of canned (high in salt). Drain and rinse canned beans and choose low-sodium versions of canned soups. Also, choose unsalted nuts and seeds.

Food Allergies and Sensitivities

Often, people with respiratory disease also suffer from food or other allergies, which can have a negative impact on both the upper and lower respiratory tracts as well as your body's overall inflammatory and immune responses. Food allergies occur when your body's immune system overreacts to a food or substance that it *mistakenly* perceives as a threat.

Food allergies can range from mild to life threatening (anaphylaxis). The most common manifestation of food allergies is *chronic rhinitis* or inflammation of the mucus membranes in the nose, but food allergies can also impact the respiratory system in the form of shortness of breath, cough, tightness in the throat or difficulty swallowing, wheezing, airway obstruction and swelling of the lips, face and tongue.

You may be surprised to hear that 90% of all dietary allergies are caused by 8 foods. These include eggs, milk and dairy products, peanuts, tree nuts (pecans, walnuts, almonds), fish, shellfish (shrimp, crab, lobster), wheat or gluten and soy. People with specific food allergies may also react to similar or related foods. The severity of symptoms is generally associated with the amount of the allergen ingested, but as a general rule, it is best to eliminate the offender from your diet completely.

Gas and Bloating

Excessive gas and bloating can also create problems for people with respiratory disease. Again, think about everything that takes up space in your stomach, increasing the intra-abdominal pressure. Remember, your body doesn't care if this increased pressure is due to solid, liquid or gas. If gas or bloating is a problem for you, consider limiting or avoiding gas-producing foods and carbonated beverages. As an alternative, you can try using an enzyme-based, gas-reducing food additive like Beano.

What the FODMAP???

Research has shown that something called the "low FODMAP diet" improves symptoms of Irritable Bowel Syndrome (IBS) such as gas and bloating. FODMAP stands for Fermentable Oligosaccharides (fructans and galactans), Disaccharides (lactose), Monosaccharides (excess fructose) and Polyols (sugar alcohols such as mannitol and sorbitol). In other words, FODMAPs are a group of small-chain carbohydrates commonly absorbed in the small intestine that could cause discomfort if you exceed your trigger threshold. Everyone has a different threshold. If you experience gas and bloating related to your respiratory disease, a low FODMAP diet may be helpful to you even if you have never been diagnosed with IBS.

Here are some high-FODMAP foods to limit or avoid:

High Lactose: Cheese: Ricotta and Cottage Cheese; Beverages: Cow's Milk; Yogurt, Ice Cream, Custard.

Excess Fructose: Vegetables: Jerusalem Artichokes, Asparagus, Sugar Snap Peas, Sun-Dried Tomatoes; Fruit: Apples, Cherries, Figs, Mangos, Pears, Watermelon; Sweeteners: Agave, Honey, High Fructose Corn Syrup; Alcohol: Rum.

High Fructans: Vegetables: Artichokes, Garlic, Leeks, Shallots, Onion, Onion and Garlic Salt/Powders; Fruit: Dried Fruit, Nectarine, Persimmon, Plums, Prunes, White Peaches, Watermelon; Grains: Rye, Wheat, Barley, Chicory Root (Inulin); Teas: Chamomile, Fennel and Oolong.

High Galactans: Legumes (Beans), Pistachios, and Cashews.

High Polyols: Vegetables: Cauliflower, Sweet Corn, Mushrooms, Snow Peas; Fruit: Apples, Apricots, Blackberries, Nectarines, Pears, Peaches,

Plums, Prunes, Watermelon; Sweeteners: Sorbitol, Mannitol, Maltitol, Isomalt, Xylitol (Sugar-Free Gum/Mints).

If these symptoms sound like you consult a *FODMAP-experienced* nutritionist who can help you design a low-FODMAP diet. Another option is to experiment on your own with FODMAP elimination and re-introduction to determine your personal FODMAP threshold.

Fiber

Fiber is a form of carbohydrate that regulates blood sugar, promotes the passage of food through your system and may help prevent many chronic diseases. Constipation can increase intra-abdominal and intra-thoracic pressures, making breathing more difficult. We should try to eat 20 to 30 grams of fiber per day in the form of whole grains, fruits and vegetables and beans. If gas and bloating are a problem for you, low-FODMAP, fiber-rich foods include oatmeal, oat bran, brown rice, rice bran, chia seeds, flax seeds, strawberries, blueberries, oranges, spinach and quinoa.

Gastroesophageal Reflux Disease (GERD)

Often, people with respiratory disease also suffer from another condition called Gastro-Esophageal Reflux Disease (GERD). Many are not even aware of it (silent reflux) but GERD can actually cause, trigger, or worsen their respiratory condition (and vice versa). Often, once GERD is discovered and treated, their respiratory condition improves as well.

GERD is caused when acid backs up from the stomach through the lower esophageal sphincter, damaging the esophagus, throat, and possibly, the airways and lungs. While the most common symptom of acid reflux is heartburn, GERD can also cause a sore throat, bitter taste in the throat and mouth, chest discomfort (non-cardiac) and abdominal pain, as well as many "respiratory" symptoms such as coughing, wheezing, and shortness of breath.

The exact cause of acid reflux and GERD is unknown but several factors contribute to or exacerbate the problem, including obesity, diet (particularly fried, fatty, spicy, and acidic foods like citrus and tomatoes), caffeinated beverages and chocolate and mint flavorings. Drinking alcohol or cigarette smoking can also exacerbate the problem, as can certain medications including antihistamines, calcium-channel blockers, nitrates and theophylline, sometimes used to treat pulmonary disease. Consuming large meals or eating close to bedtime can also contribute to GERD. Finally, GERD can result from other medical conditions like hiatal hernia, pregnancy, rapid weight gain and diabetes, in particular.

Lifestyle modifications for people suffering from GERD include weight loss, dietary modifications (e.g. avoiding known triggers, eating smaller and more frequent meals and not eating or drinking close to bedtime). Quitting smoking and minimizing alcohol intake are also recommended.

Elevating the head of your bed by 6-12 inches (or sleeping with a wedge) can help reduce symptoms. Pharmaceutical and surgical options are also available but are beyond the scope of this text and should be discussed with your physician.

Nutritional Supplements

First and foremost, it is important to understand that vitamins and minerals are best utilized if you get them as part of a healthy, balanced diet. Be sure to include foods rich in antioxidants such as vitamin C (red pepper, green pepper, papaya, strawberries, broccoli, oranges, cantaloupe), vitamin E (sunflower seeds, almonds, hazelnuts), selenium (Brazil nuts, tuna, sardines, salmon, sunflower seeds), and carotenoids (carrots, sweet potatoes, red peppers, spinach, cantaloupe, kale, collard greens, mango, butternut squash).

If you have difficulty getting all of your vitamins from food, you may want a little extra insurance. Choose a complete, *age-adjusted* multivitamin that contains 100% of what you need but not more and take it either once daily or every other day. Avoid the MEGA-vitamins as too much of a good thing will either wind up in your toilet bowl in the form of very expensive urine, or worse, cause harm. Speak to your physician or nutritionist about the right type and dose of supplements for you.

As we discussed, calcium, vitamin D and magnesium are important for bone health, especially if you are at increased risk for osteoporosis or have been on steroids. Again, do not go above the recommended daily dose and when taking a calcium supplement, be sure that it also contains vitamin D and magnesium. If your vitamin D level is low (get it checked!), you can supplement with additional vitamin D_3.

Finally, a high-quality omega-3 fish oil supplement is beneficial due to its cardio-protective and overall anti-inflammatory properties. Choose a fish oil supplement with a decent dose of both eicosapentaenoic acid (EPA) and docosahexaenoic acid (DHA). Don't be fooled by supplements that boast 1000 mg of fish oil; you need to make sure you are getting actual DHA and EPA as other oils are sometimes included in the 1000 mg of "fish oil." Compare labels and choose supplements with high amounts of these two beneficial fatty acids.

For herbal and homeopathic remedies, I strongly suggest carefully evaluating them on a case-by-case basis with your doctor, nutritionist or pharmacist, especially as they may affect your medical condition and medications.

At this time, let's take another look at that Italian dinner from our earlier example and examine the individual components of the meal and their impact on breathing. First and foremost, the meal contains *a lot* of carbs, so for the next several hours, your body will be working harder to blow off the excess CO_2 produced.

Appetizers: Shrimp Cocktail and Fried Calamari

This patient had two appetizers. Now, on its face, the shrimp cocktail was not a terrible choice (unless, of course, you're allergic to shrimp). Shrimp are high in protein, and low in carbohydrates and fat.

Then, he and his wife "shared" an order of fried calamari. Now, I don't know about you, and I certainly don't want to make any assumptions, but when some people say that they shared an appetizer, the person they were sharing it with ate only three pieces of calamari and they ate the rest (sheepishly raises hand).

The calamari is fried, making it high in saturated fat and calories and most people eat calamari lathered in tomato sauce (more about that later). It might have been a better choice to forget that second appetizer or to opt for a green salad with vinaigrette dressing.

Bread: Italian Bread with Olive Oil

Most Italian breads served in restaurants are made using white (bleached) flour. As a result, much of the nutritional value you might get from a whole grain or whole wheat bread has been eliminated. In addition, bread consists primarily of carbohydrates, which can increase the production of carbon dioxide, causing or increasing shortness of breath. Olive oil is an example of a monounsaturated (heart-healthy) fat, so if your goal is to gain weight, more power to you. However, if your goal is to lose weight, then at 9 calories per gram, olive oil is not the best choice, so you really have to be careful with portion size. A better choice would have been to ask for whole wheat bread or avoid the bread altogether.

Main Course: Chicken Parmesan

Chicken is a better choice than beef or veal. However, once breaded and fried, it becomes much less healthy. Add tomato sauce and cheese, and you could do much better. A better choice would have been grilled chicken or fish (e.g. branzino, salmon).

Side Dish: Linguini with Tomato Sauce

Again, white (bleached) pasta has a high carbohydrate load with very little nutritional benefit, increasing the production of carbon dioxide (and shortness of breath). I don't know about where you live but most restaurants in NYC serve about a pound of pasta per serving, which is well above the recommended serving size. Whole-wheat pasta has more nutrients than bleached. If you suffer from GERD, the acid in the tomato sauce will definitely create problems. A better choice would have been a side of spinach sautéed in olive oil.

Dessert: Tiramisu

Tiramisu is high in calories, saturated fat, and sugar. But, let's face it. It's also super delicious. Eat desserts like this sparingly, and if you have to have one, share it with someone. A better choice would have been a bowl of mixed berries (without the whipped cream).

Alcohol: 2 Scotch and Sodas

In addition to acting as a central nervous system depressant (i.e. hampers your breathing), alcohol also negatively impacts how you metabolize the meal. The bubbles in the soda will take up space in your stomach, increasing intra-abdominal and intra-thoracic pressures and resistance against the diaphragm, making breathing more difficult. A better choice would have been to have one drink and eliminate the bubbles.

Caffeine: Cappuccino

Caffeine is a central nervous system stimulant. It increases your heart rate, blood pressure and respiratory rate, potentially making you more short of breath. A better choice would have been a decaf cappuccino or coffee with low fat or skim milk.

I'm sorry. I promise that my goal is not to take the enjoyment away from your night out, but I hope now you at least understand why you weren't able to breathe well at the end of your five-course meal.

Let's look at this scenario from one more angle—math. The average person takes in approximately 6 liters (6000 milliliters) of air per minute. When your stomach was empty, let's say that you were able to take in 500 milliliters of air per breath. In order to get 6 liters per minute of air, you would have to breathe at a rate of 12 breaths per minute (500 x 12 = 6000). Now, sitting in that lovely Italian restaurant with your stomach completely full, you may only able to take in 250 milliliters per breath, so in order to get your 6 liters of air, you would need to take 24 breaths per minute (250 x 26 = 6000). And if you really overate, maybe you're only taking in 150 milliliters of air per breath. That would mean taking 40 breaths per minute (150 x 40 = 6000). In other words, you're panting like a dog.

So, next time you can't understand why it's so hard to breathe after a meal, think back to this chapter and remember that the shortness of breath you're experiencing is most likely a combination of mechanical (the diaphragm not being able to contract downwards), chemical (increased production of carbon dioxide), and emotional (increased anxiety as your breathing worsens) factors.

Tips for Eating for Pulmonary Patients

- Avoid large meals. Instead of 2-3 large meals, eat 5-6 smaller "*feedings*" per day. In other words, eat frequently (roughly every 2-4 hours, depending on your goals) but in small quantities so that the food you eat doesn't take up all of your available breathing space.
- If decreased appetite is an issue or you are trying to gain weight, drink at the end of your meal as opposed to before or during.
- If you are trying to lose weight, drink water before and during your meal.
- During the meal, pace yourself and use pursed-lip breathing.
- If shortness of breath is an issue, use your rescue inhaler 15 minutes before eating.
- If you use supplemental oxygen, wear it while you eat.
- If secretions are a problem, clear your airway before eating.
- Keep a food diary to monitor the impact of different foods on your breathing and energy levels.
- Eat mindfully, not mindlessly.

Keeping a Food Diary

Write everything down that you eat and drink including time, how much you ate and how you felt afterwards. Take note of food's impact on your shortness of breath and energy levels and record those in your diary. Observe how your body reacts to different foods with respect to type, amount and timing. Keeping a diary will also make it easier for your physician or nutritionist to understand your needs and offer the most effective advice.

I often say: "if you want to change your life, you have to change your life." That is, if you want to see significant results, you need to make a significant change. Changes that don't require any discipline will not lead to the changes that you want. A coordinated effort and a little willpower will help you find and stick with a nutrition program that fits *your* lifestyle and *your* health needs.

CHAPTER 10
EMOTIONS

Courage doesn't always roar. Sometimes courage is the quiet voice at the end of the day saying, 'I will try again tomorrow.'"
– Mary Anne Radmacher

Like yin and yang, your physical and emotional wellbeing are intimately related to each other. In addition to the physical impact on your body, living with a chronic illness can have a profound impact on your emotional health and wellbeing, as well as your overall quality of life—and vice versa. This is especially true when the primary symptom of that that illness is the inability to breathe. Conversely, emotional factors such as stress, anxiety, and depression can have a profound impact on your *physical* health and wellbeing. In many cases, these negative emotions can increase your symptoms or even *cause* disease.

The good news is that like many of the relationships we discuss in this book, the reverse can also be true. Emotions such as peace, love, and happiness (yes, my parents, Mel and Sherry were hippies) can have a profoundly *positive* impact on your physical wellbeing, and in many cases, help reduce your symptoms and minimize their impact on your life and *prevent* disease.

"Whether you think you can, or think you can't—you're right."
– Henry Ford

I often encounter people during some of the worst times of their lives. Perhaps they have been newly diagnosed or maybe they are experiencing an exacerbation or progression of their existing disease or some other setback in their lives. This can be difficult to cope with from both a physical and emotional perspective. After all, not being able to breathe can be incredibly stressful, anxiety provoking, *and* depressing.

Life with a chronic illness definitely can (and will) have its ups and downs. But, guess what. So can life *without* a chronic illness. Ups and downs are a natural part of being human. Regardless of who you are, some days will shine brighter than others and other days, things will get dark. Sometimes, everything in your life will seem perfect and sometimes, well, quite simply, they will suck. The key is not to get stuck in "Suckville."

"When we are no longer able to change a situation, we are challenged to change ourselves."
– Victor Frankl

Please don't think that I am minimizing your situation. I am *not*. I also understand that what I am saying is easier said than done and sometimes, no matter what you do, it can be hard to dig yourself out of that hole. That's when it's time to ask for help, whether it be from your doctor or other health care professional, friends or family members, clergyman or clergywoman, dog, cat, bird; or whomever or whatever it may be that helps pick you up when you're down.

This chapter was particularly challenging for me. I kept going back and forth between a physiology-based, science-intensive chapter, a pop-psychology feel-good pick-me-upper, and a locker room halftime speech. In the end, I decided to incorporate a little of each, with the purpose of motivating you, giving you some helpful tips and sending you back out on the field, feeling ready to kick some butt.

I have also decided to share some of my favorite quotes with you; particularly those in which, I, myself find comfort or motivation or that otherwise inspire me when I am being faced with my own personal challenges, of which there have been many. Hopefully, you will find them helpful as well. If not, feel free to cross mine out and write in your own.

***"The only constant in life* is change."**
– Greek Philosopher, Heraclitus of Ephesus

The Greek philosopher, Heraclitus of Ephesus, lived from 535 BC-475 BC and is best known for his doctrine on change being central to the universe. This goes hand in hand with "this too, shall pass," attributed to either Persian Sufi poets or King Solomon of the bible depending on your source.

"This, too, shall pass."
– Persian Sufi Poets or King Solomon

Both of these quotes remind us that change is inevitable and that we should not find it surprising when things in our lives shift, be it for better or for worse. In fact, we should be more surprised if and when things stay the same. Another piece of advice to be gleaned from those messages is to try to embrace the change, roll with the punches, soak in life's beautiful moments and push through the challenges because *nothing* lasts forever; again, for better or for worse.

As always, this chapter is *not* is a substitute for a personal consultation with your doctor, mental health counselor or any other health care professional. With that in mind, let's talk about stress, ba-by!

Stress, Anxiety and Depression

For most of us, the word "stress," is synonymous with words like pressure, anxiety, depression, loneliness or one of many other *negative* emotions. However, contrary to what many people believe, not all stress is bad. In fact, stress can serve as a powerful motivator in our lives.

Eustress (i.e. good stress) occurs when we are motivated in a *positive* way in response to a certain *stressor*. This positive response allows us to focus our attention and perform better under pressure or to deal with a challenging or dangerous situation. In contrast, *distress* (i.e. bad stress) is what most people typically think of simply as "stress." Left unchecked, this *negative* stress can be overwhelming and lead to a whole host of physical and emotional problems.

Everyone experiences some degree of stress in their lives that will fluctuate in terms of intensity and duration. While the severity of these negative emotions will vary from person to person, repeated or prolonged exposure to stress; or even brief periods of very high levels of stress can be a major threat to your happiness and your health. Prolonged or repeated feelings of stress can contribute to conditions like anxiety and depression, which can become chronic problems in themselves and lead to all kinds of negative physical, emotional, mental and behavioral consequences.

For those already living with a major health problem like respiratory or cardiovascular disease, long-term stress can have especially severe consequences if the person doesn't recognize the problem and take steps to address it. Let's take a look at some of the potential manifestations of stress, as well as some things you can do about them. There is likely some overlap among categories, which can make dealing with your emotions particularly challenging, especially when you are already living with a chronic illness.

As an example, having COPD, IPF or PH can unquestionably cause you to experience low energy or fatigue. However, stress, anxiety, or depression can also cause fatigue and these physical and emotional manifestations can play off of each other, which is even more of a reason to address these issues head on. You don't have to make all of these changes at once. However, a little effort in each area can go a long way towards improving your physical health, emotional wellbeing and quality of life.

Here are some of the more common *physical, emotional, cognitive and behavioral* manifestations of stress, anxiety and depression:

Physical Manifestations

Although it can be tempting to blame your cardiopulmonary condition for every physical symptom you experience; stress, anxiety, or depression, can also be contributing factors, if not the cause. In addition, because negative emotions and physical symptoms often go hand-in-hand, identifying whether your emotional state is the cause or the effect can quickly turn into a classic case of "which came first: the chicken or the egg." As an example, are you experiencing shortness of breath and fatigue due to your respiratory condition or because of stress, anxiety or depression? Or is it a combination of factors? This is where an open conversation with your physician *and* a comprehensive physical examination can be useful. Some of the more common *physical* symptoms that can be associated with stress, anxiety and depression include the following:

- Low energy, fatigue
- Dry mouth or difficulty swallowing
- Headaches, jaw clenching or teeth grinding
- Body aches and pains or increased muscle tension
- Chest pain, rapid heartbeat, or palpitations
- Nervousness, shaking, cold, clammy hands/feet
- Upset stomach, diarrhea, constipation, nausea, or dizziness
- Insomnia or other sleep disturbances
- Frequent colds or infections
- Loss of sexual desire, drive, or ability

Emotional Manifestations

Emotional signs of stress can be harder to quantify since each person has a different threshold for stress, anxiety, depression and other negative emotions. Sometimes, these emotions may be less noticeable or for some people, may seem like a "normal" part of your everyday life but I can assure you, *they are not.* Some of the more common *emotional* symptoms associated with stress, anxiety and depression include the following:

- Anxiety
- Irritability, anger, agitation, or hostility
- Lack of motivation or focus
- Depression, generalized sadness
- Feeling overwhelmed, loss of control, or the need to control
- Restlessness, difficulty relaxing or quieting your mind

- Avoiding others, loneliness, or isolation
- Low self-esteem or feelings of worthlessness

Cognitive Manifestations

Like emotional signs of stress, mental or cognitive difficulties can often be hard to pinpoint. While external factors often contribute to negative emotions, our mental state both affects and is affected by recurrent feelings of stress, anxiety and depression. In other words, stress can be caused by internal factors such as negative self-talk, pessimism, and perfectionism, among others. However, these factors can also be reinforced by constant stress, anxiety, and depression creating a persistent cycle of negativity. Some of the more common *mental* or *cognitive* symptoms associated with stress, anxiety and depression include the following:

- Constant worrying
- Anxious, racing thoughts
- Memory problems, forgetfulness and disorganization
- Inability to focus, concentrate
- Poor judgment
- Pessimism or seeing only the negative

Behavioral Manifestations

Finally, stress can also trigger changes in your personal preferences, habits and everyday activities. Friends or family members may notice or comment on your new or uncharacteristic behavior. Some of the more common *behavioral* symptoms associated with stress, anxiety and depression include the following:

- Anger or emotional outbursts
- Nervous behaviors, nail-biting, fidgeting, pacing
- Abusing alcohol, drugs, or tobacco
- Changes in appetite, overeating or not eating enough
- Procrastination, neglecting responsibilities
- Sleeping too much or too little
- Exercising less often
- Social withdrawal

What Can We Do?

According to British philosopher, Alan Watts, "By replacing fear of the unknown with curiosity, we open ourselves up to an infinite stream of possibility. We can let fear rule our lives, or we can become childlike with curiosity, pushing our boundaries, leaping out of our comfort zones, and accepting what life puts before us." For our purposes, I take this quote to mean that we can't alleviate stress-related *symptoms* unless we address their underlying cause. With this in mind, here are some ideas of ways to reduce your stress level.

Get Educated!

Fear of the unknown can very often worsen or intensify whatever situation you are dealing with. When it comes to finding out about your medical condition, everybody is different and has different levels of "wanting to know." For me, personally, it is almost always better to find out as much information as I can, and what I can do to deal with the problem head-on.

This can be especially important for people living with a chronic illness. By learning as much as you can about your disease, its associated symptom, and available treatments, you will be in a better position to make decisions regarding your care and your life. In addition, this understanding can help you gain a greater sense of control, reduce your day-to-day stress, and contribute to your overall sense of wellbeing.

"Knowledge is the antidote to fear."
– Ralph Waldo Emerson

In an ideal world, your doctor or his staff would have all the time in the world to sit down with you and explain your diagnosis, test results, and treatment options. However, while many medical professionals make patient education a regular part of their practice, we know that others simply don't have the time to do this for each patient.

Thankfully, there are many other resources that can help you find the information you need. As I have mentioned from the start, there is *a lot* of information on the Internet. To be sure that the material you are finding is both relevant and accurate, I would suggest *starting* with some of the official disease-related foundations and associations like the American Lung Association and their Better Breathers Clubs, the Pulmonary Fibrosis Foundation and the Pulmonary Hypertension Association, among others.

I would also like to invite you to view my *Ultimate Pulmonary Wellness* Webinars. During these 1-2-hour-plus webinars, I discuss key components of optimal disease management as well as having the honor of having many of the tippy-top specialists in their respective fields as my guests.

The Ultimate Pulmonary Wellness Webinar Series can be found online at:

www.PulmonaryWellness.com/Webinars

Get Support!

Humans are, by nature, social creatures and we know that social support plays a huge role in shaping our emotional health and enhancing our quality of life. Chronic harmful emotions like stress, anxiety and depression can feel exponentially more oppressive when we are dealing with them in isolation. We all have busy lives, but spending time with loved ones can significantly improve your emotional state, mental health, and physical wellbeing.

That being said, while the support of family and friends is extremely important, this can sometimes present its own challenges. As an example, you may not feel comfortable sharing certain aspects of your disease with them. You may feel like they will not be able to understand your situation or you may not want to burden them with your concerns.

This is where a support group can be a tremendous help. By belonging to a group in which, people have the same or similar condition, you will come to realize that you are *not* alone. You will have the opportunity to interact with people who are going through similar struggles, and who knows? You may even be able to serve as a resource to someone else in need. Whether in-person, by telephone, or online, support groups can help you learn from the experience of others and share your own in return.

The UPW Facebook Group can be found online at:

www.facebook.com/groups/UltimatePulmonaryWellness

Work It Out!

Making exercise a priority can elevate your mood, boost your physical, mental and emotional health, help lower stress, and reduce feelings of anxiety and depression. Regular exercise can also reduce blood pressure and further elevate your mood through the release of endorphins, our body's natural painkillers and mood enhancers. Focusing on improving your health through increased activity can also give you a greater sense of control in your life.

Eat Well!

What you eat can have a tremendous impact on your mood, energy level and ability to deal with stress, anxiety, and depression. Many different factors contribute to the what, when, and why we eat, and being more conscious of these factors can help to improve your physical health and your emotional wellbeing.

To help combat negative emotions, avoid refined or processed foods, particularly foods high in simple carbohydrates, sugars, and saturated fat. Instead, eat a balanced diet with plenty of fresh vegetables and fruits, lean, high-quality proteins, and healthy fats and oils.

Similarly, avoid alcohol, which is a central nervous system depressant and limit stimulants like caffeine (e.g. coffee, teas, soda), which, in addition to making you feel jittery and potentially more short of breath, can increase your feelings of stress, anxiety, and depression.

Breathing, Meditation and Mindfulness!

Breathing exercises and meditation have been used for centuries as calming techniques. There are many ways that you can incorporate breathing, meditation, and mindfulness exercises into your life. There are specific classes in meditation and pranayama (yogic) breathing, as well as methods like Yoga, Tai Chi, or Qigong that can improve your breath control, while calming and quieting your mind. You can also take a few moments each day to sit quietly, simply focusing on your breathing while clearing your mind of distractions.

There are three particular resources that I absolutely *love* and want to share with you. One is a book/CD called: "The Healing Power of the Breath" by Richard Brown, MD. In it, Dr. Brown teaches about the role of stress, anxiety, and depression in health and disease and offers solutions to these problems in the form of various meditation techniques. It also comes with a CD to lead you through the meditations and breath work.

Second, is the Qigong for Pulmonary Health program, created by Brian Trzaskos, PT, LMT, CSCS, CMP, MI-C, Founder and Director of the Institute for Rehabilitative Qigong and Tai Chi (www.IRQTC.com).

Here is a meditation that Brian created, specifically, with the pulmonary patient in mind:

- Sit comfortably with your feet flat on the floor, hands in your lap, and spine as long and tall as possible.
- Tuning into your body, feel your feet connected to the ground and your bottom resting in the chair. Take a moment to simply notice your breathing, without trying to change it. Just witness the process by which your body breathes naturally. Even if it feels labored or uncomfortable, trust that your body is doing

its absolute best to seek balance. Simply let your breath do whatever it does naturally as we cultivate the confidence in our body's inherent wisdom.

- When you feel relaxed and settled, slowly begin to lengthen and deepen your exhalations by breathing in through your nose and out through pursed lips. Inch by inch make each successive exhalation a little deeper while remaining comfortable and relaxed. After each exhalation, imagine guiding the inhalation deeper into your abdomen by allowing your belly to expand. You may notice that slightly longer and fuller exhalations often promote deeper inhalations.
- As you continue to breathe slowly and deeply, imagine exhaling toxins out of your lungs. You may visualize these toxins as brown or black smoke. However, feel free to choose something most suitable to you. Remember to stay in a comfortable and relaxed state as you slowly clean your lungs of toxins. After a few rounds of cleansing exhalations, while inhaling through the nose imagine breathing back into your lungs a soft white light. Visualize this white light filling your lungs with each successive inhalation, finding its way into every nook and cranny of your body. Imagine this white light carrying with it the capacity to heal and strengthen your lungs and respiratory system.
- Continue to exhale through pursed lips and imagine breathing out toxins from your lungs and also your abdomen. With each successive breath visualize yourself cleansing your whole body of waste products and toxins. And on each successive inhalation feel and imagine a soft white light filling your entire body. Silently repeat to yourself, "toxins out, healing in," "toxins out, healing in," "Toxins out, healing in."

In addition to the above, there are many meditation and mindfulness apps online that can guide you through some of these techniques. The one that I currently like best are "Calm," an app that focuses on breathing, meditation, mindfulness and sleep, "Insight Timer," that focuses on exploring techniques, recovery and sleep; and "OMG Meditate," which also has many guided meditations with various focus groups in mind.

Be Kind (to yourself)!

Besides exercise, eating well, and meditation; make time to relax and treat yourself to some of the things that you enjoy and that make you feel good about yourself. Take a friend to dinner, take your dog for a walk, play with your children or grandchildren, listen to music, get a massage, manicure or pedicure, knit, needlepoint, color or paint, dance, or whatever else it is, that makes you happy.

Think Positive!

Optimism and/or pessimism can have a major impact on your physical, mental, and emotional health. I realize that maintaining a positive attitude is sometimes easier said than done, but people who have a positive attitude often have a greater ability to deal with stress. Taking steps to reframe your attitude and negative self-talk will prepare you to cope more effectively with stressful situations and to fight off anxiety and depression.

Take steps to surround yourself with positive influences. If you're constantly being assaulted by cynical people, negativity, or rude comments; or depressing or anxiety-provoking TV shows or other media outlets, you will have a much harder time breaking the cycle of negativity.

"The most important decision is to be in a good mood."
– Voltaire

LOL!

There's a reason why we often call laughter the best medicine. Laughter has the ability to lower our stress level, decrease anxiety, and reduce depression. Laughing can relieve both physical and emotional tension in our bodies, reducing the level of stress hormones in the blood and stimulating the release of endorphins, relieving pain and promoting healthy immune function.

Finding a way to laugh productively in stressful or depressing circumstances may seem challenging at first, but, like anything, it gets easier with practice. Make humor an intentional part of your life. In the end, the method doesn't matter as much as trying to lighten the mood, whenever possible.

We need more kindness, more compassion, more joy, and more laughter. I definitely want to contribute to that.
– Ellen DeGeneres

Seek Professional Help

Finally, if despite your best efforts, you're still having a hard time coping with your emotions, you might consider seeking professional help. Psychiatric professionals, counselors, and religious leaders offer different types of therapies to help get you back on track. There's no shame in asking for help when you need it and no shame in trying medication when appropriate and under the care of your physician.

Making the Change

Living with a chronic respiratory disease is not easy and can trigger negative emotions such as stress, anxiety, and depression, both in the moment and over the long-term. One of the ironies is that when we're feeling stressed, anxious, depressed, or angry, we often engage in the exact opposite behaviors that we should. We decrease our participation in healthy activities like exercise and increase our participation in unhealthy behaviors like eating poorly or using tobacco.

Please understand that I am not minimizing your feelings or saying that it will be easy. I recognize and appreciate the gigantic emotional toll that living with a chronic illness can have on a person's life, especially one in which shortness of breath is a primary symptom. The good news is that you *do* have the power to change and there *are* things that you can do to minimize your symptoms and improve your life.

"You're braver than you believe and stronger than you seem, and smarter than you think."
– Christopher Robin

CHAPTER 11
PREVENTION OF INFECTION

"An ounce of prevention is worth a pound of cure."
– Ben Franklin

Living with a chronic illness, particularly a respiratory condition can significantly compromise your immune system, making you more susceptible to picking up a bug, catching a cold or developing an infection or exacerbation of your existing pulmonary condition. Patients often report getting sick once, twice, three times or more over the course of a given year and whether it is a cold, the flu, pneumonia, or an exacerbation, it *always* seems to settle in the chest.

Frequent illnesses or exacerbations, or even one bad one, can impact the progression of your disease and its associated symptoms. For this reason, it is crucial not only to take care of yourself when you get sick, but also, that you take specific measures to PREVENT yourself from getting sick in the first place.

One thing that is important to realize is that even if you do everything right, you *still* might get sick anyway. However, our goals are to decrease the probability of your getting sick in the first place, increase your ability to fight off and recover from illness, and reduce the severity of that illness, when you do get sick, minimizing its impact on your life.

How We Get Sick

At the most basic level, disease is caused by pathogens. The most commonly encountered pathogens are bacterial, viral, fungal or parasitic in origin. The most common routes of transmission include: airborne or inhaled, direct contact, indirect contact or contact with a contaminated surface, sexual contact, contact with infected blood or body fluids, and the fecal-oral route.

Viruses and bacteria cause the majority of respiratory infections and unless you are living in a bubble, you will likely come in contact with one (or a million) of these on a daily basis. They are introduced to our bodies, through the mucus membranes of the eyes, nose, and mouth, either by inhaling them or by touching or coming into contact with a contaminated surface, and then touching your face.

We are also exposed to, and come into contact with spaces, surfaces and objects that are exposed to and contacted by many people on a daily basis. Anything that is touched by many people, many times each day has a greater chance of being contaminated with bacteria, viruses and other pathogens.

Depending upon the type of organism and the surface on which they are found, some viruses and bacteria can live outside the body for up to 24 hours. Whether or not you actually get sick depends upon the specific virus or bacteria and the status of your own immune system.

Please understand that I am not trying to scare you into hermetically sealing yourself in bubble wrap. What I am trying to do is raise your awareness of everyday potential exposures so you can better protect yourself against them. Here are some suggestions on how to do that:

"Don't Patchke Your Face"

My Grandma Peppie used to say: "don't patchke your face." Patchke is a Yiddish word that means to play around or fiddle with. It was good advice then and it's good advice now. As I mentioned previously, pathogens are introduced to our bodies, through the mucus membranes of the eyes, nose, and mouth. So don't fiddle.

Wash your Hands (a lot)!

This goes hand in hand (pun intended) with "don't patchke your face." Frequent hand washing is your single best defense against introducing viruses or bacteria into your system. Most of us know (or should know) that we're supposed to wash our hands before we eat, or after we use the bathroom. However, that's not adequate, particularly for someone living with a pulmonary disease. You really need to be washing your hands each and every time you come in contact with a potential source of infection.

Also, to be clear, when we talk about hand washing that does not just mean a quick rinse. *Effective* hand washing means using soap and water, and rubbing your hands together *vigorously*, for at least 30 seconds. Keeping in mind that you initially turned the water *on* with dirty hands, turn it off using a paper towel so that you don't contact those germs again. The same goes for the bathroom door.

Antibacterial Gels/Creams/Lotions

If you don't have access to soap and water, carrying a small bottle of anti-bacterial gel, cream, or lotion can come in "handy". Some people may argue against using anti-bacterial products, on the grounds that they kill the good bacteria along with the bad. While this may be true to some degree, I would still choose using an anti-bacterial gel over walking around with the common cold or pneumonia on my hands, just waiting for an opportunity to enter my mucus membranes.

Antibacterial Sprays and Wipes

Remember also that objects or surfaces that you come in contact with may not be cleaned frequently (or ever), and therefore, may be contaminated with a whole host of pathogens. For this reason, it is well worth your time and effort to spray or wipe them with disinfectant before you use them. As just one example, when you go to the supermarket, wipe down the shopping cart before leaning all over it or putting your food inside.

At the Pulmonary Wellness & Rehabilitation Center, we have dispensers with anti-bacterial foam for our patients and staff. We also wipe down every machine in between each and every patient. The last thing we want is for people to get sick *at a wellness center.*

Protect Your Home

When you return home after a day out, you carry with you all of those nasty 'bugs' (bacteria and viruses) that have latched onto you and your belongings over the course of your day. You can help minimize their impact and reduce the likelihood of contaminating your home by taking a few precautionary measures.

First, as previously mentioned, wash your hands as soon as you walk in the door, and even better, take a shower. Change out of your dirty "outside clothes", and into your clean "inside clothes", and swap outside shoes for inside shoes or slippers.

When visitors enter your home, ask them to take similar precautions. Well, maybe not the shower part, but they can certainly take off their coats in the hallway, remove their shoes at the door, and wash their hands when they arrive. This is even more important when children are visiting. Since children are much more likely to come in contact with dirt, viruses and bacteria, it would be to *everyone's* advantage if they have an extra set of clothes to change into and immediately wash up, especially after they've been playing outside.

Protect Your Property (O_2 Equipment and Supplies)

If you use oxygen, it is important to protect all of your supplies and equipment including the tank or concentrator itself as well as all of the accessories including tubing, masks and cannulas. All of the bugs that can travel with you on your clothes and your property, can also travel on your oxygen equipment. Be aware of where you place your equipment both at home and when you are out and wipe it down frequently with an antibacterial wipe, especially when returning home. With respect to your cannula or mask, be sure to place them on something clean when not in use and wipe them down if they have been sitting for a while. I can't tell you how many times, I have seen people's cannula hanging on the floor or thrown into their bag unprotected. If you keep it in a plastic bag, wipe it down BEFORE you put it in the bag and...wipe down the bag.

Be Aware of Your Surroundings

Equally important to being vigilant at home is minimizing your risk of exposure when you are out. As mentioned previously, this is particularly important when you are in public places that are regularly frequented by a lot of people.

Again, think about how many people's hands touch the handrails on escalators or stairs, equipment at the gym, door handles or push buttons. I'll give you a hint. It's *a lot*. And the poles on buses and subways are virtual petri dishes for every disease known to man and probably a few yet-undiscovered ones as well.

As both a gambling man (and a health-care professional), I'm particularly aware of the "disgusting factor" at a casino. How many hands have touched those slot machine arms, the chips or the huge stack of cash you're hoping to put in your pocket?

And then…there's the doctor's office. Now, that's a whole 'nother ball of bacteria (and viruses). Besides the obvious, *coming-in-contact-with-a-high concentration-of-sick-people-in-one-place*, how often do they clean the tables and chairs? And what about that annoying pen on a chain? Or even the magazines? If in doubt, don't be afraid to confirm that the area and equipment have been disinfected. While this may seem like an imposition on the staff, as healthcare professionals they should appreciate your concern and understand that it's better to be safe than sorry (or sick). As Ronald Reagan said: "Trust, but verify."

Dining Out

Dining out comes with its own unique risks of exposure to bacteria and viruses at every stage of the process, from the food preparation, to its distribution, to its consumption. Every person, from the host or hostess, to the chef, to the server, and every item from the table, to the menus, to the plates and utensils, to the food itself is a potential source of contamination. A weak link in any of these areas can increase your risk of exposure and illness. I don't know about you, but if I go into a restaurant and my server is sick, I simply excuse myself, leave a tip, and make it my business to get the heck out of there as fast as I can.

Other Factors

You can't make the whole world germ-free. However you can do your best to protect yourself. Here are some other suggestions:

Stay Away From Sick People

That may sound overly simplistic, or even harsh in some cases, but it is both completely true and very important. Of course, we understand that you want to see your friends and family, but trust me, if your children are sick (or even your grandchildren), it is much better to take a rain check—for *everyone.* As someone with a chronic pulmonary disease, a cold for you is not the same as a cold for someone with a healthy immune system, and as heartbreaking as it might be to skip the visit; you really have to look at the big picture. If that visit lands you in the hospital, it doesn't do anyone any good.

Stay at Home When You're Sick

Rule Number One: if you are sick, just stay home! We are conditioned to believe that we should never, ever, *ever* miss a day of work. However, that is a surefire way to prolong your illness and *maximize* its spread to as many people...and places...and surfaces as possible.

At the Center, our policy is if you are sick, you stay home, no if's, and's or but's. This applies to patients and staff alike, even if you feel well enough to exercise or come to work. Again, the last thing we want is for you to get sick at a wellness center or for you to get someone else sick at a wellness center (or anywhere else).

Get the Flu Shot

Many people ask whether or not they should get the flu shot. While there is no single best answer for everyone, the Center for Disease Control recommends that everyone 6 months or over should get the flu shot annually. This is especially true for people over 65, or anyone with a medical condition that could compromise their immune system such as respiratory and cardiovascular disease. However, individual cases will vary depending on age, level of risk, medical condition(s) and doctor preference, among other factors, so to be sure, check with your personal physician.

Get the Pneumonia Vaccine

Like the flu shot, there is no single best answer for everyone and again, individual situations will vary, so to be sure, please consult your personal physician. Up until recently, it was generally recommended that people over 65, or anyone with a medical condition that could compromise their immune system, get a one-time, single-dose vaccine, called the "pneumococcal polysaccharide vaccine 23 (PPSV23). However, based upon the findings of a large clinical trial, that recommendation has changed. At the time of this writing, the CDC recommendations are as follows:

- In addition to a single dose of PPSV23, at-risk individuals, 65 years of age or older, should also get a dose of the pneumococcal conjugate vaccine 13 (PCV13), which provides protection against community-acquired pneumococcal pneumonia and other *pneumonia* infections.

- People who have never had the pneumonia vaccine should get the PCV13 FIRST and get the PPSV23 six to twelve months later.
- People who have already had the PPSV23 should also have the PCV13 as long as it has been at least one year since their initial vaccination with PPSV23.

Get Enough Rest

Sleep affects every system of the body, from the immune to the endocrine, to the cardiovascular and pulmonary, and every other system in between, to some degree or another. Lack of sleep or not getting enough overall rest can have a negative impact on your body's immune system, lowering your body's resistance and its ability to defend itself against bacteria and viruses. While most guidelines recommend between 7 and 9 hours, the exact amount of sleep we need varies from individual to individual.

Don't Smoke!

Cigarette smoking is one of the worst possible things you can do to your body. As if causing heart disease, lung disease, cancer and complications during pregnancy weren't enough, smoking cigarettes also lowers your body's immune function and increases your chances of developing an infection or exacerbation. So just don't do it.

Avoid Triggers

In addition to bacteria, viruses and other pathogens that can make you sick, there are other substances and conditions that can act as "triggers." These triggers can cause a range of symptoms including irritation of the eyes, nose or throat; cough, tightness in the chest, shortness of breath, or inflammation of the airways and lungs. All of these mechanisms of the inflammatory process can make you more susceptible to developing an illness or exacerbation.

Triggers can be more universal in scale like air pollution or weather, or they can be more personal and individualized like coming in contact with a strong odor or cigarette smoke. Here are some of the more common triggers that can particularly affect people with respiratory disease:

Indoor Allergens

Indoor Allergens include things like dust, mold, cockroaches and roach droppings, and pets and animal dander, among others. Symptoms can include, coughing, sneezing, stuffy or runny nose, as well as itching, burning or tightness in the ears, eyes, nose, mouth, throat, or chest. In these situations, it is crucial to eliminate the source of exposure, whenever possible OR to remove yourself from the exposure. This can be difficult in each of the above situations, for various reasons. However, the longer time that you are exposed and the more intense the exposure, the greater the chances are and the greater the potential damage that you are likely to experience.

Outdoor Allergens

Outdoor Allergens include things like pollen, trees, grass, weeds, and mold, among others. Similar to indoor allergens, symptoms can include, coughing, sneezing, stuffy or runny nose, as well as itching, burning or tightness in the ears, eyes, nose, mouth, throat, or chest. These allergies will likely be greatest from the spring through the fall and your best bet is to avoid exposure as best you can. If you are exposed, treat it similarly to exposure to a virus or bacteria by washing your hands frequently and changing your clothes and showering when you come back home. Saline eyewashes may be beneficial as well as nasal and oral saline rinses. Pay attention to the local pollen and other allergen counts and speak with your doctor about any over the counter or prescription medications that might be helpful.

Pollution

People living in more industrialized, densely populated urban areas will likely be more exposed to pollution than those that live in areas that are more rural, sparsely populated and less industrial. Air pollution includes various gases, ozone in particular, smoke, haze, smog, and ash, among others. Depending upon where you live and the type of pollutants, the conditions can change seasonally, daily, or even over the course of a single day. In the case of environmental incidents or emergencies, conditions can change rapidly and dramatically.

Pollution will typically be worst on hot, humid days in the city. The Environmental Protection Agency (EPA) reports the Air Quality Index (AQI), which measures air quality based upon 5 pollutants: ground level ozone, particle pollution, carbon monoxide (CO), sulfur dioxide (SO_2), and nitrogen dioxide (NO_2). It is ground-level ozone and airborne particulate pollution that pose the greatest threat to humans (and animals), particularly, those in high-risk groups, like respiratory disease.

Check the AQI at www.airnow.gov if you plan on being outside for any significant period of time. On days when the air quality is poor (greater than 100), consider limiting your time outdoors and avoid strenuous activity. Since ozone is generally higher in the afternoon and evening, try to organize your day accordingly, going out in the morning instead of later in the day.

Occupational Exposure

Certain jobs, hobbies and other activities will increase your chances of being exposed to one or more substances that can cause or worsen your respiratory condition. These include toxic chemicals and other irritants such as smoke, asbestos, dust, dirt and debris, among many others. Ideally, you will be able to avoid this type of work but if this is not possible, be sure to be aware of and *use* maximum personal protection equipment (PPE) for the type and level of risk involved. This includes protective masks, gowns, gloves as well as any other specific protective gear for the particular task at hand.

Weather

Many people are affected by weather, particularly, either by heat and humidity or by cold, dry air. When it is hot and humid outside, the air seems to be thicker and heavier. As a result, people with respiratory disease are forced to work harder with each breath in order to move air in and out. When it is particularly hot and humid, try to go out early in the morning before the sun is at its strongest or in the late afternoon or evening, after the sun has begun to go down.

On cold, dry days, the airways can become narrower due to bronchoconstriction and spasm of the smooth muscle lining the airways. Ask your doctor if you can take your rescue inhaler or nebulizer about 15 minutes *before* going out. Also, cover your nose and mouth with a scarf, mask or other product that can help warm the incoming air.

Other Exposures

There are other exposures that are more personal, individual, or situational in nature and while I can't possibly name them all, here are a few examples:

- Cigarette (or other) smoke
- Perfumes, colognes and other scented oils or lotions
- Air fresheners, candles and incense
- Construction
- Cleaning products
- Other

Again, I am not trying to scare the bejeezus out of you. However, in many cases, depending upon the type, severity, and degree or intensity, one exposure can sometimes be enough to cause a problem, especially if you are already compromised in one way or another; to trigger inflammation or an exacerbation, or to get you sick. So, please take the extra time and effort to protect yourself and your loved ones.

Don't Shake Hands or Kiss Hello and Goodbye

While it may be customary to shake hands when you meet someone, it is definitely *not* in your best interest. Now, I'm not trying to be gross, but in most cases, you really have no idea when that person last washed their hands. In this situation, social mores have to take a back seat to your health. The same goes for the hello and goodbye kiss and doubly so for the double kisses. You get the idea.

You can try using an alternative greeting: say "N*amaste*", bow, wave, or salute each other. Hell, throwing up a gang sign (joke). Or, you can simply let people know that you don't shake hands. Whether or not you tell them the reason is up to you, but it could be a good teaching opportunity and a chance to educate others about your condition. The choice is yours. No pressure.

Throw Tissues Away Immediately After Use

This one may seem obvious, but I can't tell you how many people I see blowing their nose and then putting the dirty tissue back in their pocket, purse, up their sleeve, or in their bra (or what I like to call: "Grandma's tissue box")...and, don't even get me started on the handkerchief! I don't know who thought of this brilliant idea, but do you really want to save that stuff for later? Besides being a treasure trove of bacteria, they're just gross. So don't use one.

Avoid Confined Spaces

Whenever possible, avoid spending prolonged periods of time in small, enclosed spaces with poor ventilation. Try to stay in large, open, well-ventilated areas with lots of fresh air and where close contact with others is less intense.

As an example, airplanes are one of the worst possible places when it comes to the transmission of illnesses for a whole host of reasons. There are lots of people, in close proximity to each other. The air is re-circulated around the cabin and the surfaces are rarely disinfected. This makes it very easy for bacteria or viruses to travel from person to person, on surfaces or through the air. Although not quite as bad, the situation is similar in small offices, elevators, or other enclosed areas.

Suit Up

Let's face it. Regardless of how well we attempt to prepare ourselves for every possible condition, we are all going to encounter situations in which we have no control over our environment. When all else fails and you find that you cannot control the environment or those around you, more extreme measures must be taken. Suit up. When we know we are going to be in a hostile environment, wearing a mask and/or gloves can be an effective last-ditch effort to avoid exposure.

Seek Medical Attention Sooner Rather Than Later

By now, you should realize that I believe in the "better safe than sorry", "err on the side of caution," and "an ounce of prevention..." schools of thought. When in doubt, seek medical attention *sooner rather than later*. As I have mentioned on many occasions, a cold is not the same for me as it is for you or someone with a respiratory disease; and a day or two, and sometimes even a few hours, can be the difference between preventing and minimizing the impact of a problem versus really getting in trouble. Many doctors will give their patients a prescription for antibiotics and/or steroids to keep on hand for if and when they do get sick.

Other Suggestions

Recently, I asked the members of my Ultimate Pulmonary Wellness Facebook group to share some of their own personal practices for preventing infection. Here are some of their suggestions:

- Use antioxidant vitamins, minerals and herbs; particularly, vitamin c, zinc, Echinacea, and green teas
- Use immune-boosting products like "Airborne" or "Emergen-C"
- Use gut health-enhancing probiotics
- Use nasal rinses and throat gargles
- Use an air filter/purifier

CHAPTER 12
AIRWAY CLEARANCE

"Out, damned spot! out, I say!"
– Lady Macbeth

Written with gratitude to my Co-Author, ***Marion Mackles, BS, PT, LMT***

Everyone has mucus. It is one of the many defense mechanisms in our body's arsenal that protect us against infection and other *un*-pleasantries. In fact, if Lady Macbeth were a chest physiotherapist, she may well have been known for another quote: "Out, damned snot!" Before we discuss how to minimize and mobilize the secretions (mucus) that may accumulate in your airways as a result of your disease, it will be helpful for you to have a basic knowledge of what mucus actually is and what mucus actually does.

Take a breath in through your nose. Congratulations! You have just inhaled a small sample of the many thousands of tiny organisms and a varied array of particulate matter that we breathe in each and every day. When we breathe in through the nose, the air goes through its first warming, filtering, and humidifying process. If you are a mouth breather, the respiratory tissues will have to handle the job on their own, further down the respiratory tract.

The mucous (different than mucus) tissues or *membranes* that line the nasal cavity have a sticky surface that helps trap debris, like flypaper. There are also tiny hair-like structures called *cilia* that help move the air and mucus through the sinus cavity to prepare it for its journey into the lungs, the GI tract; or to be expectorated. Our airways and lungs perform a similar filtration process as air passes through them. This filtration system is called the "*mucociliary escalator*," or "*mucociliary transport system.*"

The Airway Swamp

The airways leading into the lungs are lined with epithelial cells that protect the airways and lungs. These cells are loosely square-shaped and have thousands of cilia. Scattered throughout the epithelial cells are mucus-producing goblet cells. This is where I start to draw a picture in my mind of a swamp. The cilia float in a thin mucous fluid that is slightly thicker than water and a thick layer of mucus that rests on top of the cilia. That's the stuff that traps debris; which I like to picture as bugs in the swamp; that are stuck to the top scummy layer.

Under all of that, we have clear, crisp water in which our cilia (swamp plants) move back and forth in a wave-like motion. This wave-like motion pushes the mucus up through the airways, millimeter by millimeter to the throat, where it is either swallowed or expectorated (coughed out). If it is swallowed, the stomach acids destroy any organisms that may be living in the mucus. In addition, to swallowing or expectorating, some smaller particles of mucus are expelled as vapor when we exhale. This process automatically takes place every second of every day, whether we have a pulmonary condition or not.

Just like the ecosystem of a swamp, any alien intruder or other irritant can throw this well-coordinated system out of balance. In response, the goblet cells start *overproducing* mucus to help fight whatever irritant or foreign invader may be present. In addition, goblet cells from the lower layers can break through to the upper layer, overpowering the ciliated epithelial cells. At this point, we lose the wave action of the cilia, and the sluggish goblet cells take over the swamp. This delicate transport system can also be affected by other factors like scar tissue or paralyzed cilia (from cigarette smoking or exposure to environmental toxins), temperature, and humidity.

AIRWAY CLEARANCE TECHNIQUES

When it comes to airway clearance techniques, patients often ask, "which method works the best?" and the answer is always the same: "it depends on the individual." Every person is *at least* slightly different with respect to his or her anatomy and physiology, disease process and progression, level of conditioning, lifestyle, etcetera, and etcetera. For that reason, it will often take some trial and error to figure out what will work best *for you*, but at some point, you have to take the first step. Starting somewhere and doing *something* is always better than doing nothing!

When it comes to the techniques themselves, you have many options available to you, including the many devices on the market such as positive expiratory pressure (PEP) devices, oscillating PEP devices, valves that alter sound wave frequencies, and vests, among others. There are also manual chest therapy techniques that require a second person to assist you. However, before we get to those, let's talk about some of the techniques you can do on your own and without spending a penny. These techniques can be used on their own *or* in tandem with one of the various devices to make the treatment even more effective.

I usually recommend performing the airway clearance techniques two to three times per day. The most important (and effective) times are in the morning, shortly after you wake up and in the evening about an hour or so before going to bed, *not* immediately before bed. Sometimes, it can take a while for the mucus to come up and we don't want your sleep to be disturbed by coughing. Many of the positions people sleep in are also natural drainage positions (which we will discuss later). Did you ever notice that when you wake up in the morning, one of the first things you do is clear your throat, cough, or even hack up some sputum? This is the perfect time to take advantage of Mother Nature by using one of the clearance techniques for maximum benefit.

In the evening, you want to clear out your lungs of whatever may have accumulated during the day. These times can also be coordinated with your medications. Some techniques work well 5–15 minutes after taking your bronchodilator. Vests and some of the other devices can be used *while* nebulizing to help the medications go deeper into the lungs. But, before we get too far ahead of ourselves, let's look at the techniques.

Active Cycle of Breathing Technique (ACBT)

The *Active Cycle of Breathing (ACBT)* consists of a series of different breathing patterns that help loosen and mobilize mucus for expectoration; i.e. huffing, coughing, or in some cases, "hacking out" the mucus. ACBT requires no equipment and can either be performed sitting in a chair or in one of the postural drainage positions. For most sessions, I prefer not to have patients leaning back in the chair. When you lean back and rest on a surface, you are inhibiting ribcage movement and airflow to that part of the lungs. Instead, sit straight up with your feet flat on the floor. Please check with your physician before trying these techniques and if possible, schedule a session with a chest physical therapist or health professional trained in ACBT. If this is not possible, begin your practice slowly with the basic cycle.

A. Breathing Control or Relaxed Breathing (1 minute)

Settle into a relaxed, gentle, pattern of breathing in through the nose and exhaling quietly (not forced) through pursed lips, although some people teach this with an open mouth. If you have difficulty breathing in through your nose, breathe in through pursed lips. This step will relax the airways and accessory muscles and can also help alleviate anxiety. Breathing control should always be done before a huff (more on this in a moment).

B. Deep Breathing or Thoracic Expansion (3–5 breaths)

While taking a slow, deep, breath in, expand your lower ribs, allowing air to fill your chest. Don't force it! You may want to do this in front of a mirror placing your hands on your lower ribs when you are first learning this technique. Once your lungs are full, hold your breath for 2–3 seconds. If you are uncomfortable with breath holding (or prone to pneumothorax), you can skip this step. Then, sigh your breath out through pursed lips, allowing your ribcage to deflate slowly, like an accordion.

C. Huffing or Forced Exhalation (1–3 breaths)

Huffs are a form of forced exhalation. To do this, open your mouth wide with a relaxed dropped jaw. Imagine that you are trying to steam up your glasses before you clean them.

The basic pattern is ABAC, which equals one cycle:

A. Breathing Control or Relaxed Breathing (1 minute)

B. Deep Breathing or Thoracic Expansion (3–5 breaths)

A. Breathing Control or Relaxed Breathing (1 minute)

C. Huffing or Forced Exhalation (1–3 breaths)

I recommend repeating the cycle until you have expectorated, but no more than 3 times so you don't wear yourself out. Often, a patient will become very productive about a half hour to an hour *after* ACBT.

There are two different types of huffs:

C1: Lower Airway Huff:

Take a small to medium breath in and give an extended huff out. The lower airway huff clears secretions from your lower airways.

C2: Upper Airway Huff:

Take a long, slow, deep breath in and give a quick huff out. The upper airway huff clears secretions from your upper airways.

If you choose to do both types of huffing, separate them by 1 minute of ***Breathing Control*** in between. Depending on your ability, or what works best for you, the cycle can be extended (e.g. ABABAC1). You can also perform several cycles (e.g. ABAC1/ABAC2/ABAC1). In this case, the pattern would be:

Cycle 1:

A. Breathing Control or Relaxed Breathing (1 minute)

B. Deep Breathing or Thoracic Expansion (3–5 breaths)

A. Breathing Control or Relaxed Breathing (1 minute)

C1. Lower Airway Huff (1–3 breaths)

Cycle 2:

A. Breathing Control or Relaxed Breathing (1 minute)

B. Deep Breathing or Thoracic Expansion (3–5 breaths)

A. Breathing Control or Relaxed Breathing (1 minute)

C2. Upper Airway Huff (1–3 breaths)

Cycle 3:

A. Breathing Control or Relaxed Breathing (1 minute)

B. Deep Breathing or Thoracic Expansion (3–5 breaths)

A. Breathing Control or Relaxed Breathing (1 minute)

C1. Lower Airway Huff (1–3 breaths)

Depending on the therapist, there may be slight variations in the methods and techniques used. However, as always, the individual protocols should be adapted to match the needs and abilities of the patient.

Controlled Cough

I like my patients to complete every chest clearance session with a 3-tier controlled cough. We are not talking about hard, forceful coughs that tighten the throat and irritate the tissues. When done properly, coughing is one of the most effective clearance tools.

Sit with your feet flat on the floor, shoulder-width apart. Place both hands on your abdomen, pressing slightly inward like a girdle. Take a slow, deep breath in through your nose and hold for 2–3 seconds. Then, bending forward, simultaneously give 3 small, short, staccato-type coughs in a single breath while continuing to apply pressure to your abdomen. If you need to repeat this process, perform 1 minute of breathing control/relaxed breathing before continuing.

Splinted Cough

If you need more support, you can wrap your arms around your abdomen or hug a pillow or towel. This is particularly helpful following thoracic or abdominal surgery. If this is the case, place the pillow or towel over the incision site and squeeze for added support and to reduce pain. This is also effective for anyone who might have musculoskeletal or orthopedic issues or osteoporosis that might be prone to spontaneous rib fractures, including people who have been on steroids for prolonged periods or at a high dosage.

Postural Drainage

Postural drainage consists of 12 different positions that use gravity to help mucus drain from the various lung segments into the larger airways, where it can be expectorated. I recommend holding each position for 5–15 minutes; and some specialists recommend even longer. Like everything else, you just have to try it and learn what works best for you. Some people need to incorporate all the positions into their daily routine, while others only need to use one or two regularly.

Many patients benefit from leaning over a table while sitting or standing, performing deep breathing exercises. Some hang over their beds; or use a tub chair or bench. Sitting in the shower, they lean forward while splinting their arms on their legs or on the wall in front of them, while doing deep breathing or ACBT. Many people find that the steam from the shower helps loosen their secretions, making it easier for them to expectorate.

Postural drainage techniques are best done with ACBT. Many patients also use PEP devices to loosen the mucus even more while in these positions. Some people benefit from taking their bronchodilator 5–15 minutes *before* postural drainage and any nebulized steroids or antibiotics about 30 minutes to an hour *after* postural drainage.

NOTE: Do not eat for an hour before your postural drainage treatment.

In addition to the drainage positions alone, healthcare professionals can also use percussion (or cupping), vibration, and shaking when performing chest therapy and teach these techniques to family members or caregivers. In some positions, the patient can percuss himself/herself or use a small handheld vibrator. You can also buy handheld cupping devices that are specifically designed for chest therapy (not musculoskeletal treatments). As always, please find a trained health care professional to teach you and your caregivers the proper techniques and adaptations to suit your particular situation.

Percussion (Cupping)

Contrary to what some of you may have experienced, percussion or cupping does not involve hitting or slapping the hell out of somebody with an open hand. *When done properly*, this technique should *not* be painful at all. To perform cupping, gently cup your hand, clapping the chest wall in a rhythmic pattern, alternating hands. Instead of a slap, you should hear a hollow, popping sound and feel the flow of air passing between your hands. To protect the skin, the patient should wear a thin layer of clothing like a t-shirt or hospital gown. Keep in mind that you are *not* trying to bang the mucus out. What you *are* doing is vibrating air molecules to shake the mucus loose.

Vibration

Vibration involves placing a flat hand firmly over the focal area; typically over the ribcage. Keeping your own trunk stable, stiffen your arm and hand, causing it to shake. The patient should take deep breaths in through the nose and out through the mouth, with vibration being performed during exhalation. This technique along with cupping is extremely effective in helping to mobilize secretions.

Always end your sessions with some good deep breaths and controlled coughing (or huffs, or both). Again, please check with your doctor before beginning any chest therapy program, especially if you have any musculoskeletal or orthopedic issues, cardiovascular conditions, GERD (acid reflux/acid stomach), or hemoptysis (blood in your sputum).

Now that we have covered treatments you can do at home, mostly without help, and without purchasing anything, let's move on to the world of valves and other gizmos aka airway clearance devices.

Airway Clearance Devices

Incentive Spirometer (IS)

Many people ask about the incentive spirometer and may even have one hanging around from a previous hospital stay, particularly, following a thoracic, abdominal or other surgical procedure. These plastic devices use plastic balls or a plunger-type indicator to provide a patient with visual feedback for inhaled airflow and volume. Using this device can help prevent atelectasis, pneumonia, and other pulmonary complications caused by prolonged bedrest, anesthesia, and/or pain medications. An incentive spirometer helps to clear secretions by visually cueing a person to take in a greater volume of air, opening up the lungs more fully.

Some of our patients find that using an incentive spirometer helps them to take a few deeper breaths either prior to postural drainage or at the end, before performing a controlled cough. Anything that helps you take a deeper breath or mobilize secretions is a good thing!

The incentive spirometer comes with a list of settings of normal volumes based on age and gender. Start with a setting that is just *slightly* above the highest amount that you can currently perform, gradually increasing the volume as your lungs improve. We instruct our patients to take a slow, deep breath in through the nose and gently blow out through pursed lips. Then put the mouthpiece in your mouth with a tight seal and slowly inhale. When you get to your peak, hold the breath for 1–3 seconds and then let the air out gently. Some clinicians will ask you to blow the air out into the apparatus. I ask my patients to take the mouthpiece out and exhale through pursed lips.

Usually, people are instructed to repeat the process 10 times in a single sitting, but patients often start to fatigue their diaphragm, making this an exercise in futility. Instead, repeating only 3 cycles at a time, allows you to focus on the process, slowing things down and making it more effective, without becoming exhausted. The first time allows you to get a feel for the exercise, the second lets you make any necessary adaptations, and the third time is for the win! However, do not stress too much about performing an exact number of breaths or exhaling with or without the mouthpiece. Instead, try to focus on properly executing the *inhalation* through the mouthpiece. Always end your sessions with some deep breathing and controlled coughing (or huffs, or both).

POSITIVE EXPIRATORY PRESSURE VALVE

The PEP (Positive Expiratory Pressure) valve is not used as often but has been around since the 1970s. Once the oscillatory PEP valves (Flutter, Acapella) became available in the 1990s, many doctors, therapists, and patients switched over. On a PEP valve, you take a deep, full breath and exhale slowly through the mouthpiece. When blowing out, the device's resistance pressure (between 10–20 cm H_2O) helps splint open the airways. This allows more air to move along the airways below the mucus to move it into the larger bronchi. Most of these devices have a manometer to ensure you are creating the right amount of pressure.

Once again, start in a comfortable seated position. Using your ACBT, perform 1 minute of breathing control relaxed breathing. This time, replace the deep breathing portion with 10 inhalations and exhalations through the PEP. Continue to follow your ACBT while substituting the deep breathing portion with the PEP device. To visualize this method, I like to think about the air flowing down the sides of airways, speeding by trapped cloud-like shapes of mucus. Then, I picture the air reaching a bulb-shaped bottom where it whips around for a high-speed return trip up the center of the airways, pushing the mucus up with it. Please note that as with all of the PEP devices, make sure that you are not puffing your cheeks, which will diminish the effects. If you find that you do tend to puff your cheeks, use one hand to hold them while exhaling.

While positive expiratory pressure makes mucus clearance easier by opening up the airways, it does not do anything to thin out or break up that hard-to-clear mucus—which brings us to oscillating PEP devices. In addition to providing positive expiratory pressure, these devices vibrate as you blow out.

Flutter Valve

The **Flutter Valve** made its US debut in late 1994 or early 1995 and is shaped like a small pipe. Inside, are a small cone-shaped funnel and a metal ball. As you blow out of the device, the ball bounces up and down, causing short spurts of intermittent positive expiratory pressure and a vibration that resonates and is amplified in the airways. The great thing about the **Flutter** is that it is small, durable, and easy to clean. However, the Flutter's success is highly dependent on proper positioning. You have to be in an upright position (preferably sitting in a chair or sitting up in bed) with your chin slightly tilted upward. The device itself must be held at a certain angle with the stem (mouthpiece) parallel to the floor at approximately 15 degrees above or below parallel.

Many of our patients have trouble consistently finding the position that works best for them or achieving a vibration. However, when this device is used properly, it works well. Generally, once you have found a position where you feel a good resonant vibration in your upper airway and hear a good flutter sound from the pipe, sit in straight position with your feet flat on the floor and head tilted up (you can rest your elbows on a table to splint open the ribcage if you need). You are ready to begin the session.

The Flutter is used in 2 stages:

Stage 1: Mucus Loosening and Mobilization

Making sure that your lips have a tight seal on the mouthpiece, take a deep breath in to fill your lungs fully (but do not force the air in). Hold your breath for 2–3 seconds, and then blow out quickly but not forcefully. Your exhalation should be controlled and longer in duration than your inhalation. Remember; do not puff your cheeks. Repeat this step 5–10 times. I often ask my patients to perform 1 minute of relaxed breathing control before repeating another 5–10 breaths through the Flutter. During the first stage, it is important to try to suppress your coughs.

Stage 2: Mucus Elimination

Inhale deeply (totally filling your lungs). Hold this breath for 2–3 seconds, and then blow out as forcefully as possible. Try to empty your lungs completely. Repeat this cycle 1 more time followed by a cough (or a huff and a cough).

It takes a while to get a feel for the apparatus and to figure out how many breaths to do in Stage 1. Be patient with yourself.

The Acapella Vibratory PEP

A few years after the Flutter valve hit the market, the **Acapella Vibratory PEP System** showed up. The original **Acapella Blue DM** (a low-flow valve

[<15L/min]) and **Acapella Green DH** (a high-flow valve [>15L/min]) are easier to use than the **Flutter**. The device consists of a body surrounding the inner works and a removable mouthpiece. The original device cannot be opened for proper cleaning and drying. Now, these original Acapella Green and Blue are marketed as single-use devices for use during an acute hospital or nursing care stay. The company now makes the **Acapella Choice** and **Acapella Duet.** Both open and can be taken apart for proper washing.

Both device versions have resistance dials to control the frequency of the vibration and the user does not have to be in any specific position for the apparatus to work. Therefore, you can use these devices in any of the drainage positions to increase their effectiveness. The Acapella Duet has a special port for a nebulizer system and a separate chamber for the nebulized medication, which wastes less medication. This device is sturdy and can be used with or without a nebulizer.

NOTE: All Acapella products can be attached to a nebulizer. Some attach directly, and some require an adapter to attach to the end of the device. When you nebulize with the Acapella, vibrations and PEP push the meds further into your airways. We often instruct our patients to wait 5 minutes after nebulizing with the Acapella, breathe in and out through the device about 3–5 times, and then cough.

After a quick search online, you will see there are as many ways to use the Acapella as there are days in the week. I find this device effective to use with **ACBT**, but I recommend switching it up so that you begin with the **deep breathing** portion. In other words, breathe in and out, slowly but strongly, through the device for 1 minute (10–15 breaths). Then, follow with **controlled, relaxed breathing** for 1 minute. Perform each step 3 times before coughing.

1. Start **deep breathing** in and out of the **Acapella** for 1 minute or 10–15 breaths—whichever comes first.
2. Switch to relaxed **breathing control** without the device in your mouth for 1 minute
3. Immediately put the Acapella back in your mouth for another round of **deep breathing** (1 minute) and **breathing control** (1 minute), followed by another round of **deep breathing** (1 minute) and **breathing control** (1 minute), for a total of 3 cycles.
4. Take a deep breath in, hold it for 2–3 seconds, and cough (or huff and cough—whatever works for you).

As with the **Flutter,** make a tight seal on the mouthpiece with your lips and keep your cheeks from puffing out. If possible, suppress your cough until the end of the third set of your relaxed breathing/**breathing control**. If you need to cough badly, try to wait until you complete your set of **deep breathing** with the Acapella device.

There is one note to make about positioning of the device. The device must always be perpendicular to your nose (when sitting parallel to the floor), or it will not work well. As long as you maintain a 90-degree angle from your face with the device, it will work in any position that you place your body. For example, if your left side is totally congested, you can lay on your right side to inhibit air from going into that side and use the Acapella to focus your drainage on the left side.

The device does not work as well when it is moist. As a result, make sure you do not put the device back together after cleaning until it is thoroughly dry. Some people buy one device for the morning and one for the night so that they always have a clean, dry instrument.

THE AEROBIKA OSCILLATING PEP DEVICE

The **Aerobika Oscillating PEP (OPEP)** device is an incredibly convenient device that actually won an award for its design. It is very portable and lightweight. It comes apart easily for cleaning and can be put back together just as easily. Like the **Acapella**, it is not position-dependent and has a resistance setting.

Like the **Flutter** and **Acapella,** the **Aerobika** uses positive expiratory pressure to splint open the airways, while oscillations thin mucus and stimulate the cilia to mobilize secretions into the upper airways where they can be expectorated.

As with all of these devices, make sure you have a tight seal on the mouthpiece, hold your breath for 2–3 seconds before you exhale into the device (we call it the "and" beat), make your exhalation 3–4 times greater than your inhalation, and keep your cheeks as stiff as possible (no puffing them out!). Again, if you find you are puffing your cheeks, use whichever hand is not holding the device to squeeze your cheeks. A manometer accessory can attach to the mouthpiece so that you have a visual gauge to determine whether you are achieving the right amount of pressure as you breathe out. The instructions for daily use from the company are also pretty easy to follow. The manufacturer suggests breathing in and out through the apparatus for 10–20 breaths followed by 2–3 "huff coughs;" repeat this pattern for 10–20 minutes until you clear.

We use the same protocol for the **Aerobika** as we do for the **Acapella**. Once again, we use the **ACBT** switched up, starting with the **deep breathing** portion so that you start with 1 minute of breathing in slowly, but strongly, through the device (for approximately 10–15 breaths), followed by relaxed **breathing control** for 1 minute. Perform each step 3 times and then cough.

The **Aerobika** can also be used with a nebulizer. Many of our patients use this device with the nebulizing system that they already own. Monaghan, the maker of the **Aerobika,** also has their own nebulizer system (the **Aeroeclipse**), which has gotten great feedback from many of our patients. Again, if you are using the device while nebulizing, I often instruct our patients to wait 5 minutes after nebulizing with the Aerobika, and then breathe in and out through the device again (about 3–5 times), and cough.

If you use these devices for nebulizing, make sure you clean them well to prevent the medication from leaving a residue. Many of our patients will buy 2 of the same model and dedicate a device for nebulizing at home and the other for clearance without nebulizing that they carry around all day. Check with your doctor or health care professional before nebulizing with any device.

As an example, you may want to nebulize with a bronchodilator or saline solution, while using the device to open your airways or thin your mucus, respectively. Once you have cleared, nebulize with your other drugs without using the device. However, if you nebulize with medications such as anti-inflammatories or antibiotics, first clear with the device and nebulize without it. This is why it's so important to speak to and train with the proper healthcare providers. It also underscores the importance of knowing the medications you are taking—what they do and why you are taking them.

OTHER CLEARANCE DEVICES

Some patients and/or doctors occasionally ask about the **Lung Flute**, which is not actually a PEP device. It works via a low-frequency acoustical waveform produced when air is blown through the mouthpiece and over a long reed inside the device. This low-frequency wave travels to the lower airways and changes the viscosity of the mucus (making it thinner). The Flute's larger size makes it harder to carry around. It is easy to clean and comes with several months' worth of reeds. However, it can be difficult for people with weak hands or joint pain to change the reeds.

To use it, take a breath in before quickly and firmly inserting the mouth-piece and blowing into the Flute (as if you are gently blowing out a candle) for 20 sets of 2 breaths. You will hear the reed vibrate, but you will not feel a vibration like with the other devices. After each set of 2 breaths, rest for 5–10 seconds. When you are done, wait 5 minutes while secretions collect in the back of your throat. Then, cough for several minutes to bring up the secretions. The entire session usually takes about 5–10 minutes. Secretions may continue to collect for several hours after using the device.

Only a few of our patients use the **Lung Flute** because they complain that it fatigues them too much. Those who do best with this device are usually our younger and fitter asthma patients. Many patients will also use another device to clear after the 5-minute rest, prior to coughing. Some use the Flute in the morning to move the deeper secretions and use the Aerobika, Acapella, or another valve for their afternoon and/or night session.

There are a few other devices on the market that we do not see much in our practice, but occasionally a patient presents who uses one of them already or asks about it.

Another device is the **Quake**. It is small like the **Flutter** and is not position dependent. It cannot be used with a nebulizer. The **Quake** does have a very strong vibration on both inhalation and exhalation. However, patients struggle with the "handle" that controls the frequency of the vibrations that must be continuously manually rotated throughout the breathing part of the protocol.

For patients who can manage it, the **Quake** works well as a supplement for those who use other clearance devices but have difficulty bringing secretions up past their throat.

After using their other clearance device and coughing, they perform a minute of **breath control/relaxed breathing** followed by about 3–5 breaths in and out slowly through the **Quake** followed by another cough or huff. Reports from these patients have been positive.

This device has also helped some patients who aspirate food while swallowing. If they have the coordination and ability, I ask them to wait about 45 minutes after eating and then perform about 5 breaths in and out of the device, followed by a cough or huff. Often, they will cough up thin secretions with tiny food particles in them.

The **RC-Cornet/Curaplex VibraPEP** is another positive expiratory oscillatory device that is not position dependent, has an adjustable resistance valve, can be used with a nebulizer, and is reportedly easy to clean. It has a long, curved shape with a mouthpiece and a soft, flexible tube inside that vibrates on exhalation. I have never tried it, but word on the street is that it gets a "thumbs up."

Some patients benefit from high-frequency chest wall oscillation devices (**HFCWO**), also known as "vests." These devices involve wearing a vest or a wide wrap over the ribcage. They attach to tubes that are linked to a motor (generator). The vests fill with air, applying positive pressure to the outside of the ribcage. At the same time, the device pulses and shakes, causing air in the airways to vibrate, thinning and loosening secretions, and increasing airflow to move the mucus to the upper airways to be coughed out.

Some of our patients swear by these devices, but others hate them. Some disliked the brand they were using and eventually tried another, which they either loved or hated. **HFCWO**'s are big, heavy, and loud, making people less compliant when it comes to using them. Here's the rub: when they work for a patient, they work really well! You also can nebulize at the same time to get the medication deeper into the airways. I ask my patients who use these devices to perform relaxed breathing for a few minutes after completing their "vest" treatment, followed by 5–10 blows on a vibratory/ oscillating PEP device to remove their secretions from the upper airways.

A portable **HFCWO** showed up in the US market place about 3 years ago, which has a portable battery and handheld remote. This allows you to be mobile while receiving your treatments. Patients often switch things up to make these tools work for them. Some people will pause their **HFCWO** machine every 5 minutes and use their PEP devices for 5–10 blows. Some nebulize for part of their session and stop it every 5 minutes to huff or take some blows on their PEP devices for the duration of their session.

Other tools are now on the market such as the ***Vibralung*** Acoustical Percussor Electro-Mechanical Acoustical Airway Clearance. The manufacturer's 40-plus-page booklet explains how it works much better than I can. Basically, instead of working on a single frequency like the other vibratory/ oscillating PEP devices, it works on multiple frequencies at the same time.

The shorter the *wavelength*, the *higher* the frequency, and the *higher* the *pitch; higher pitches travel well in narrower airways, just like in the pipes of an organ. The opposite is true for wider airways.* While none of our patients use this device, the Vibralung may be worth looking into for people who might require a **HFCWO** but are unable to tolerate the pressure on their ribcage.

PUTTING YOUR DEVICE TO GOOD USE

At this point, I want to take a moment to talk about expectations. I always tell our patients that I see 4 types of results with these devices. The first type of patient is so productive that within a minute of starting to use the device, he or she starts to expectorate mucus.

The second type of person uses the device but does not produce any mucus until about 20 minutes to an hour later, at which point he or she becomes extremely productive and able to clear; some patients have to take a few extra blows on their device at that time to make sure they have totally cleared.

A third group reports that nothing happens with the device, except that they feel less symptomatic and can breathe better (e.g. coughing less at night). I instruct this type of patient to continue to use the device until his or her next x-ray and/or CAT scan. Many times, the tests will also show some improvement. I am not sure why this happens, but my professional opinion is that the device is breaking up this patient's mucus enough for him or her to get rid of it naturally.

Finally, the fourth group reports no changes in their condition. In these cases, I check with their pulmonologists to make sure there are no new occurrences in the patient's disease processes. If everything comes back negative, we look at other techniques, protocols, and devices to use either separately or together.

Other great ways to clear are using the Pulmonica (a harmonica designed for pulmonary patients), singing (a fast-paced song works well), laughing, and exercise. Anything that forces you to take deeper breaths in and longer breaths out can reduce your mucus.

SUPPLEMENTING WITH THE "P-*HUH*" METHOD

One of my favorite techniques that our patients love is the "**P**-*huh*" technique. This is hard to explain on paper, but let us give it a try. Tighten your lips like you are preparing to pop your "**P**." Take a deep breath in through your nose and hold it for a second or so. Next, push the air out of your mouth as if you want to throw it across a room, popping or emphasizing the "**P**" sound while saying "**P**–*huh*." It sort of sounds like a huff cough with an explosive "**P**" at the beginning. Once you master the initial "**P**–*huh*," you can move on to the exercise routine.

To do this, perform 3 sets of continuous "P-huh" sounds quickly and softly—as if you were reciting Shakespeare or a song from Hamilton:

1. Take a deep breath in and do as many repetitions as you can in a single breath: P-huh/P-huh/P-huh/P-huh/P-huh/P-huh.
2. Take another a deep breath in and do as many repetitions as you can in a single breath: P-huh/P-huh/P-huh/P-huh/P-huh/P-huh.
3. Take a third deep breath in and do as many repetitions as you can in a single breath: P-huh/P-huh/P-huh/P-huh/P-huh/P-huh.
4. Relax your breathing for 1 minute, then give me 3 explosive P-*huhs* with a breath between each: deep breath in, hold, and **P**-*huh*, deep breath in, hold, and **P**-*huh*, deep breath in, hold, and **P**-*huh*.
5. Take a deep breath, hold it for 2–3 seconds, and perform a controlled cough.

Some patients report that whenever they have a coughing spell or cannot clear, they just do a few explosive **P**–*huh* sounds and are able to clear.

Here is the take-home message: some techniques or devices may work exactly like the manufacturer's instructions describe or like your therapist taught you. Others may not help that much. Practice with different options to determine what works best for your body and lifestyle. Some people have to mix and match using a different device in the morning compared to at night or when they are sick.

Unfortunately, unlike in a shoe store, we cannot try on different sizes and colors or take a walk around the store to see how they fit. These devices (even the cheapest ones) are costly, so pick an option and try it for a while. Work with your healthcare professional to see how to make it work better for you. Sometimes, you may need to try a different device. Gauge your improvement not just by how much mucus you expel, but also by how you feel in general and in terms of your ease of breathing.

I personally tell my patients that you need to think of yourselves like a professional athlete, musician, or singer. It is your time to train to be the best you can possibly be and although working on your respiratory health can be hard, you have to work diligently for any of these tools to produce a positive outcome.

AFTERWORD
FINAL THOUGHTS

"Imperfection is beauty, madness is genius and it's better to be absolutely ridiculous than absolutely boring."
– Marilyn Monroe

As far as any of us knows, we only get one life to live and I'm going to fight for it. I may go down, but if I'm going down, you'd better believe I'm going down fighting tooth and nail and for every last breath. In the case of Ultimate Pulmonary Wellness, this means gathering up your army, and using every weapon and tool you have at your disposal. Your army includes your family, friends, doctors, and other healthcare professionals, among others. Your tools and weapons are your medications, exercising, eating well, managing your stress and anxiety, and taking steps to prevent infection.

For today, *try* not to focus on what you don't have or what you can't do. Focus on the things that you can do and *do them well.* If you can help someone else in the process, that's all the better. Answer someone's question, share your experience, express a few words of encouragement to someone that is struggling…and *breathe.* You are alive! Make sure you don't forget to live. I am with you. Make it a great one, my friends.

"Never, never, never, never give up!" **– Winston Churchill**

BOOK DESCRIPTION

Ultimate Pulmonary Wellness is a resource for all people living with respiratory disease including patients, their families and caretakers; and clinicians. This well-rounded guidebook is the fusion of twenty-five years of clinical practice, education and research by Dr. Noah Greenspan, board-certified clinical specialist in cardiovascular and pulmonary physical therapy; and Program Director of the Pulmonary Wellness & Rehabilitation Center in New York City. It is one of the most comprehensive works of its kind.

This brand new first edition draws together a complex variety of threads, clearly defining the key components of living well with a pulmonary disease; including the anatomy, physiology and pathophysiology of the respiratory system; the multifactorial and multi-systemic nature of breathing; the role of medicine (physician, diagnosis and treatment) in the management and prevention of respiratory disease; and the importance of lifestyle factors, such as exercise, nutrition and managing your emotions, as well as the prevention of infection; in ultimate pulmonary wellness; and living your absolute *best* life with respiratory disease.